ORTHOPEDIC NURSING

A programmed approach

ORTHOPEDIC NURSING

A programmed approach

NANCY A. BRUNNER, R.N., B.S.N., M.S.

Director, Special Projects,
Nursing Services, Mt. Carmel Medical Center,
Columbus, Ohio

THIRD EDITION

with **162** illustrations

The C. V. Mosby Company

ST. LOUIS • TORONTO • LONDON   1979

THIRD EDITION

Copyright © 1979 by The C. V. Mosby Company

All rights reserved. No part of this book may be reproduced
in any manner without written permission of the publisher.

Previous editions copyrighted 1970, 1975

Printed in the United States of America

The C. V. Mosby Company
11830 Westline Industrial Drive, St. Louis, Missouri 63141

Library of Congress Cataloging in Publication Data

Brunner, Nancy A   1939-
    Orthopedic nursing.

    Bibliography: p.
    1.   Orthopedic nursing—Programmed instruction.
I.   Title.
RD753.B78   1979   610.73'677   78-32020
ISBN 0-8016-0833-3

GW/M/M   9   8   7   6   5   4   3   2   03/C/343

Preface

■ This programmed text has been constructed to assist the student in learning the principles of nursing care of the orthopedic patient within a nursing process framework. Nursing actions are viewed as being taken to meet one or more goals that have been established by the nurse in interaction with the patient. The nurse is seen as guiding the patient in the goal-setting process on the basis of an assessment of current and past health status. The goals identified by the nurse and the patient and the actions selected to meet those goals comprise the patient's nursing care plan, which is communicated to other members of the health care team. The nursing care plan is then implemented utilizing the principles of care of the orthopedic patient. The impact of nursing actions on the patient is continuously evaluated and changes are made in the nursing care plan on the basis of that evaluation. However, many of the relationships between nursing actions and patient responses have not been confirmed by empirical research. The nursing approaches suggested in this text, and others, need to be empirically evaluated so orthopedic nursing can have a scientific basis for practice.

This program was designed to teach the student the terminology utilized in the provision and documentation of nursing care and in describing a variety of orthopedic conditions and their treatment. It is assumed that the student possesses a basic knowledge of anatomy, physiology, and medical terminology. It is also assumed that the student possesses basic nursing skills. The student will learn the principles of nursing care relevant to each of the primary methods used in the treatment of the more prevalent orthopedic conditions. After completion of the program, the student should be able to identify and apply the principles underlying the nursing care of the fracture patient and the surgical orthopedic patient. The student should also be able to recognize and apply nursing care principles that are appropriate in the care of the nonsurgical orthopedic patient.

This program is intended to reinforce and supplement classroom lecture content and thus is designed to permit classroom and clinical instructors to focus on assisting the student in the integration of principles and concepts. Since the examples of nursing care applications in the text are limited, the student will require the guidance of an instructor to facilitate transfer of knowledge gained from the text into the clinical patient care situation.

The text has been revised to incorporate changes in medical and surgical treatment and nursing care of orthopedic patients and to reflect epidemiological trends. However, technological innovations are occurring at such a rapid pace that the student must accept responsibility for supplementing the current knowledge base by individual inquiry via utilization of a variety of resources. This revised edition continues to emphasize the nursing care of the orthopedic patient and, therefore, may not provide an adequate reference on pathology or medical care. A list of readings has been included for the user desiring more in-depth information.

Nancy A. Brunner

Philosophy of orthopedic nursing

■ The patient with a condition or disease of the musculoskeletal system is cared for by applying the principles of orthopedic nursing within a nursing process framework. Each patient's needs and the nursing actions required to meet them are identified through nurse-patient interactions. Although the orthopedic patient's disease or condition generates some needs that are different from those of patients with nonorthopedic diagnoses, the nursing process and the principles of orthopedic nursing are applicable to all patients. The principles of orthopedic nursing are relevant for all patients, because the restoration and maintenance of function and the prevention of complications related to the musculoskeletal system are as essential for the nonorthopedic patient as they are for the orthopedic patient.

Standards of orthopedic nursing practice

   I. The collection of data about the health status of the individual is systematic and continuous. These data are recorded, retrievable and communicated to appropriate persons.

  II. Nursing diagnosis is derived from health status data.

 III. Goals for nursing care are formulated.

 IV. The plan for nursing care prescribes nursing actions to achieve the goals.

  V. The plan for nursing care is implemented.

 VI. The plan for nursing care is evaluated.

VII. Reassessment of the individual, reconsideration of nursing diagnosis, setting of new goals, and revision of the plan for nursing care are a continuous process.

Printed with permission of American Nurses Association, Kansas City, Missouri 64108.
Copyright American Nurses Association, 1975.

Contents

SECTION IV **PRINCIPLES OF NURSING CARE OF THE NONSURGICAL ORTHOPEDIC PATIENT**

section one

INTRODUCTION TO ORTHOPEDIC NURSING

CHAPTER 1

Joint motions

■ The terminology used to describe the movements of the joints is reviewed in this text because knowledge of these terms is essential in numerous phases of the nursing care of orthopedic and other patients. Joint motion terminology may be utilized in a nursing care plan to describe one or more specific extremity positions to be maintained or prevented. It may also be used to describe one or more specific joint motions to be allowed or restricted. That is, nursing care goals and nursing care plans may be made more precise and meaningful by using the appropriate joint motion terminology. In this chapter the joint motion terms are defined and applied to simple nursing care situations.

A
B; bend it upon itself
move it into a straight line

1 The extremities or a part of an extremity may be either moved into a straight line or bent upon themselves. The motion of straightening is *extension* and the motion of bending is *flexion*. Which part of Fig. 1-1 illustrates flexion? _____ Which part of the figure illustrates extension? _____ To flex an extremity is to _____ _____ . To extend an extremity is to _____ _____ .

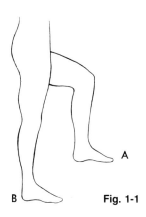

A

B

Fig. 1-1

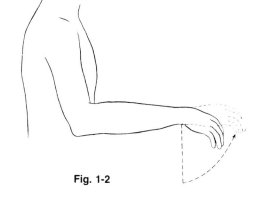

Fig. 1-2

extension

2 Motion toward a straight line by a part of an extremity is illustrated in Fig. 1-2. The motion of the hand into a straight line is _____ .

3

3 Which motion is illustrated in Fig. 1-3? _____

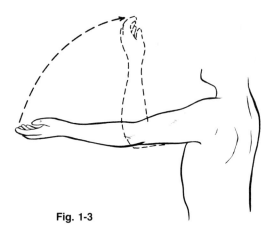

Fig. 1-3

4 Flexion and extension have been defined in terms of movement of an extremity or part of an extremity. Flexion or extension of an extremity may involve more than one joint. When the arm is extended, as shown in Fig. 1-3, which of the following joints are involved?

a, b, and d

a. wrist

b. elbow

c. acromioclavicular

d. glenohumeral

The lower leg is bent toward the femur (the extremity is bent upon itself).

5 When the leg is flexed at the knee, the lower leg is in what position in relation to the femur?

6 The extremity, or a part of it, may also be moved into *hyperextension*. *Hyper* means exaggerated; therefore, hyperextension means

extension

exaggerated _____ .

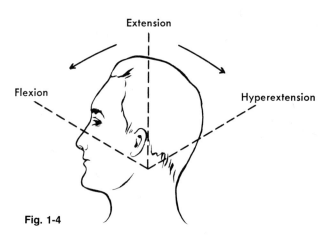

Fig. 1-4

4

7 Label the joint motions indicated *A* through *E* on Fig. 1-5.

A. _____

B. _____

C. _____

D. _____

E. _____

8 Hyperextension is a(n) (flexed? extended? exaggerated?) motion.

9 The extremities may be moved either toward or away from the midline of the body. Motion toward the midline is *adduction;* motion away from the midline is *abduction*. Motion toward the midline is (adduction? abduction?). Motion away from the midline is (adduction? abduction?).

10 The directions in which the extremities may be moved in relation to the midline of the body are _____ _____ and _____ _____.

11 After an extremity has been moved away from the midline of the body, it is said to be in an abducted position. If the extremity has been moved toward the midline of the body, it may be described as

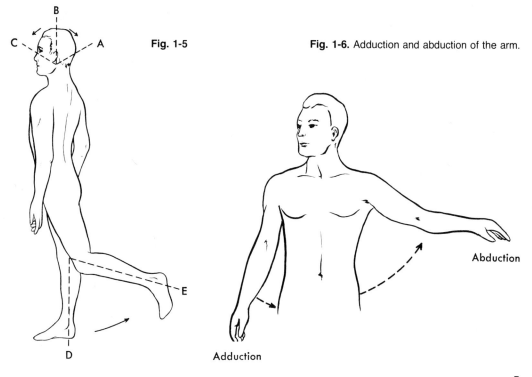

Fig. 1-5

Fig. 1-6. Adduction and abduction of the arm.

Abduction

Adduction

being in an adducted position. In order to determine the position of an extremity, the nurse should examine its relationship to the

midline of the body _____ .

abduction

12 Motion away from the midline of the body is _____ .

adduction

13 Motion toward the midline of the body is _____ .

abduction

14 Fig. 1-7 has all of its extremities in _____ .

15 What determines the difference between adduction and abduction?

The direction of the extremity motion or the extremity position in relation to the midline of the body.

16 What motions are illustrated by the directions of arrows *A*, *B*, *C*, and *D* in Fig. 1-8?

A. Adduction
B. Abduction
C. Abduction
D. Adduction

A. _____

B. _____

C. _____

D. _____

17 In addition to the motions of adduction and abduction, an arm or leg is also capable of being rotated upon its axis. This rotation is also done in relation to the midline of the body. *External rotation* is turning away from the midline of the body; *internal rotation* is turning toward the midline of the body.

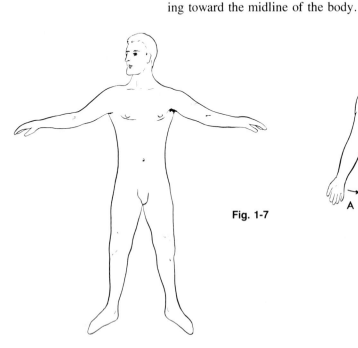

Fig. 1-7

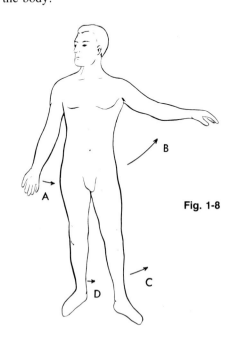

Fig. 1-8

18 Internal and external rotation are similar to adduction and abduction in that they are defined with reference to the body's

midline

_____ .

19 Internal and external rotation are different from adduction and abduction since they are defined not only in terms of the midline of the body but also in terms of turning or rotating on an _____ .

axis

20 The following table summarizes the relationships between adduction, abduction, internal rotation, and external rotation.

Type of movement	Direction of movement with respect to midline of body	
	Away	Toward
Lateral motion	Abduction	Adduction
Rotation on axis	External rotation	Internal rotation

The distinction between adduction/abduction and internal/external rotation is made on the basis of:

a. Type of movement
b. Direction of movement with respect to the midline of the body

a. _____
_____

b. _____
_____

21 Turning toward the midline on an axis is _____

internal rotation

_____ . Motion away from the midline of the body

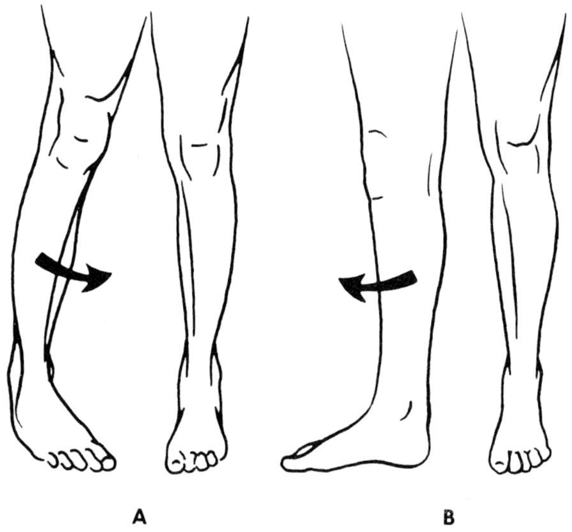

Fig. 1-9. A, Internal rotation of the lower extremity. **B,** External rotation of the lower extremity.

is _____. Turning away from the midline is _____
_____. Motion toward the midline of the body is
_____.

22 What is the difference between internal and external rotation?

23 Label Fig. 1-10 to show which arm is internally rotated and which is externally rotated.

24 The terms which have been defined can be used along with internal and external rotation to fully describe the position of the extremity. The position of the arm in Fig. 1-10, *A*, can be described as being _____, _____, and _____

_____.

25 The position of the arm in Fig. 1-10, *B*, shows the arm has been moved toward the midline of the body, which is the same as saying

it has been _____.

26 The two unique movements of the forearm are *supination* and *pronation*. Supination is the motion that brings the palm forward and makes the radius and ulna parallel. Pronation is the motion that turns the back of the hand forward and crosses the radius over the ulna.

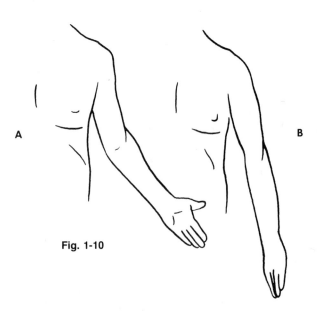

Fig. 1-10

supinated

pronated

27 The forearm may be moved into a _____ or a _____ position.

The radius and the ulna are parallel.

28 When the forearm is supinated, how are the bones positioned?

29 Describe how the palm is turned or moved in supination; in pronation.

In supination the palm is moved forward. In pronation the palm is turned away and the back of the hand is forward.

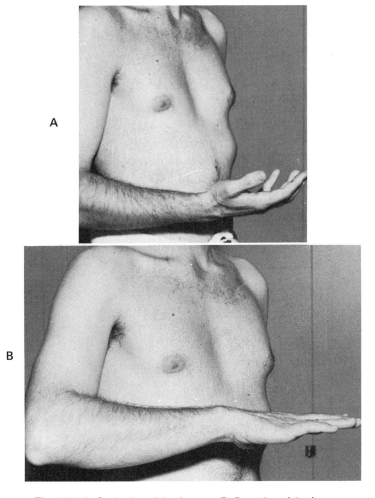

A

B

Fig. 1-11. A, Supination of the forearm. **B,** Pronation of the forearm.

30 Match the joint motion from the left column with its opposite motion from the right column.

_____ 1. Extension   a. Adduction

_____ 2. Supination   b. Internal rotation

_____ 3. Abduction   c. Flexion

_____ 4. External rotation d. Pronation

                                                e. Hyperextension

31 The lower extremity can be (flexed? extended? pronated? externally rotated?).

32 The patient is lying with her arm held tightly against her body. She has her arm _____ .

33 The nurse is going to wash the patient's perineum. To do so the nurse must move the patient's legs so they are _____ .

34 The patient has his right arm at his side. The nurse wants to check the rash in the right antecubital area. What motion of the arm would best expose the area? _____

35 The patient is sitting up in a chair. His hip and knee joints are _____ .

36 A patient who walks "pigeon-toed" appears to have his feet _____ .

37 The patient has his palm outstretched to receive a gift. The forearm is _____ .

38 When the forearm is pronated, the radius and ulna are _____ .

39 When the forearm is supinated, the radius and ulna are _____ .

40 The patient's nursing care plan indicates that his right leg is to be abducted. The patient's right leg should be moved (toward? away from?) the midline of his body.

41 The patient's nursing care plan also indicates that the nurse should do passive range of motion exercises on the patient's upper extremities. This means the nurse should move all joints of the patient's arms into all possible positions; the shoulder, elbow, wrist, and finger joints should be exercised. An arm, as a whole, can be:

a. _____

b. _____

c. _____

d. _____

42 The wrist joint can be:

a. _____

b. _____

c. _____

43 The nurse may also move the patient's forearm into

_____ and _____ .

44 The head and neck should be included in range of motion exercises unless contraindicated. The head can be _____ ,

_____ , or _____ .

45 When standing erect in a normal position the legs are

_____ .

46 The difference between adduction and abduction is determined

by _____

_____ .

47 When the patient's arm is to be positioned in abduction, it is to

be moved _____ the midline of the body.

48 An externally rotated leg is one that is rotated _____

_____ the midline of the body.

49 When the patient is described as having flexion contractures of the arms, the nurse will observe that the arms are:
a. Turned away from the midline of the body
b. Bent at the elbows and rotated toward the body

c. Positioned toward the midline of the body
d. Bent at the elbows with the forearm bent toward the upper arm

50 Joint motion terminology can be used to describe desired or re-

stricted _____ or _____ .

CHAPTER 2

Basic body mechanics

■ Body mechanics refers to the functions of muscles and joints and the application of their principles to the activities of the patient and the nurse. Body mechanics can be viewed from the perspective of the nurse or the patient. Almost all of the principles are applicable to both nurse and patient; the nurse is responsible for teaching the patient the principles of body mechanics specifically relevant to his condition. The human musculoskeletal system can tolerate only limited stress without injury, so the nurse must constantly apply the principles of body mechanics to prevent temporary or permanent injury or deformity.

functions of muscles
and joints

1 Body mechanics refers to (fluid intake? functions of muscles and joints? alimentary elimination?).

both the patient and
the nurse

2 The application of the principles of body mechanics involves (the patient? both the patient and the nurse? the nurse?).

body mechanics

3 By applying these principles, a nurse can efficiently lift and turn patients when giving care without causing injury to his or her own body. The functions of muscles and joints and the application of their principles are referred to as (body building? body maintenance? body mechanics?).

body

4 In addition to their application in the lifting and turning activities of the nurse, the principles of body mechanics are utilized in other phases of patient care. The nurse applies the principles of body mechanics when lifting or turning patients to prevent injury to the (patient? back? body?).

goals

5 The nurse applies the principles of body mechanics to the activities and positions of the patient as well as to her or his own activities. The application of the principles of body mechanics will contribute to the attainment of nursing care goals. The nurse should consider how the patient's position is related to the attainment of nursing care _____.

6 Eating is usually done in a sitting position because the gravitational flow assists the food in reaching the stomach. Thus, by placing the patient in a sitting position to eat, the nurse facilitates or permits

12

normal functioning of the patient's body. The nurse should be able to associate positioning of the patient with the appropriate nursing care goals. One such nursing care goal is to facilitate or _____ _____ .

permit normal functioning

7 From other sources you have learned that good circulation is essential for healing. The patient must be positioned so that circulation is maintained and so that his position will aid healing. The proper position of the patient in bed or chair will _____ _____ and _____ .

permit normal functioning

aid healing

8 A *contracture* is poor muscle tone resulting from inactivity. After prolonged immobility, the muscle becomes fixed in position. Body mechanics principles must be utilized to prevent contractures that would result in deformity. Application of the principles of body mechanics helps to prevent _____ that result in _____ .

contractures
deformity

9 Hypostatic pneumonia is caused by inadequate exchange in the lower lobes of the lungs. If the patient is slumped forward in a chair or bed, he cannot breathe properly. The nurse may prevent hypostatic pneumonia and other complications by utilizing knowledge of body mechanics. By practicing what he or she knows, the nurse may help to prevent _____ and _____ .

deformities
complications

10 The orthopedic patient frequently experiences pain. Orthopedic surgical procedures involve muscles and joints, and the patient's position can cause additional discomfort by stimulating muscle spasms. By altering the patient's position, the nurse may alleviate some of his pain. Application of the principles of body mechanics prevents _____ and _____ and relieves _____ .

complications; deformities

pain

11 List the five ways in which the patient benefits from the nurse's application of the principles of body mechanics.

a. The body functions normally.
b. Healing is aided.
c. Complications are prevented.
d. Deformities are prevented.
e. Pain is relieved.

a. _____
b. _____
c. _____
d. _____
e. _____

12 The nurse sets an example for the patient while performing duties. By standing or sitting properly, the nurse demonstrates the application of the principles of body mechanics to the patient. The checkpoints for the standing posture are shown in Fig. 2-1. In the correct standing posture, the head is held erect with the chin drawn in, the chest is elevated by straightening the back, which causes the sternum to be in front of the rest of the body and helps to keep the abdomen flat, and the feet are placed apart but parallel with no internal or external rotation of the legs. The checkpoints of the correct standing posture are the h_____ , c_____ , b_____ , a_____ , and f_____ .

head; chest; back
abdomen; feet

13 To set a good example for patients, the nurse must control properly the five checkpoints of the body. They are: _____ , _____ , _____ , _____ , and _____ .

head
chest; back; abdomen; feet

14 To stand straight, the head is held _____ with the _____ in.

erect
chin

15 The back is held _____ ; this elevates the chest so that the _____ is _____ of the rest of the body.

straight
sternum; in front

16 When the back is held straight, the abdomen is _____ .

flat

17 The feet should be placed (apart? close together?) and (externally rotated? pointed straight ahead? internally rotated?).

apart
pointed straight ahead

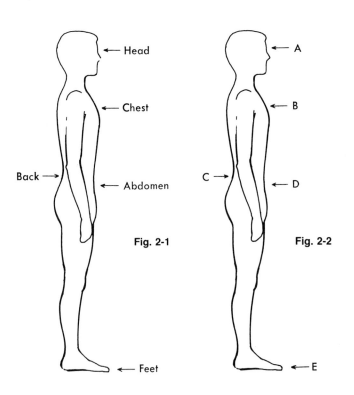

Back → — Head

— Chest

— Abdomen

← Feet

Fig. 2-1

← A

← B

C → ← D

← E

Fig. 2-2

18 In Fig. 2-2 label the checkpoints of the standing posture.

A. Head
B. Chest
C. Back
D. Abdomen
E. Feet

A. _____

B. _____

C. _____

D. _____

E. _____

19 An improper sitting position contributes to general fatigue. The standing position checkpoints may be utilized for the sitting position by also checking the flexion of the hips and the knees. The hips and the knees should be flexed at right angles.

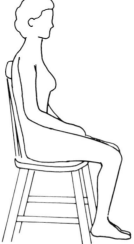

Fig. 2-3. Correct sitting posture.

20 Which part of Fig. 2-4 demonstrates the correct sitting posture? _____

B

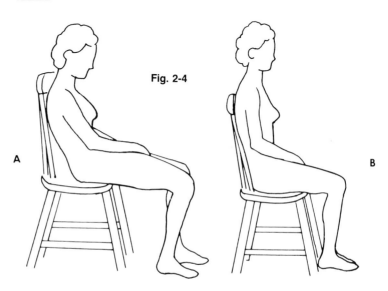

Fig. 2-4

A

B

15

21 In the correct sitting position, the hips and knees should be flexed (at any angle? at right angles?).

at right angles

22 The checkpoints for the correct sitting position are:

a. Head
b. Chest
c. Back
d. Hips
e. Abdomen
f. Knees
g. Feet

a. _____
b. _____
c. _____
d. _____
e. _____
f. _____
g. _____

23 Regardless of the position assumed, the posture should be relaxed, not stiff, to prevent additional muscle fatigue. A military posture cannot be held indefinitely and is very uncomfortable. Improper posture and bad body mechanics place abnormal stress on the weight-bearing joints. Abnormal stress on the weight-bearing joints is thought to be a factor in the development of joint diseases such as osteoarthritis. By application of the principles of body mechanics to posture and activities, the nurse can prevent the development of joint _____ and/or _____ .

disease; injury

24 To prepare to lift a load or patient, face the object and stand close to it. To facilitate lifting, the nurse should _____ the object to be lifted and be (far away from it? close to it?).

face

close to it

25 The standing posture should be checked prior to lifting and adapted by flexing the knees. The nurse must remember to hold the back straight and to use the leg muscles. The leg muscles can be utilized most effectively by _____ the knees and holding the back _____ .

flexing

straight

26 Get ready to lift by contracting the muscles. Remember that it is usually easier to pull an object than it is to push it. Just before lifting, _____ the muscles.

contract

Fig. 2-5. A, Correct lifting posture, with knees flexed and back straight. **B,** Incorrect lifting posture.

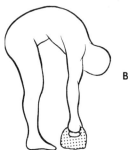

A

B

16

27 The nurse should not hesitate to seek assistance when lifting an object or patient. If other personnel are not available, mechanical equipment should be used. The amount of assistance needed is determined by the patient's ability to move and, in part, by motion restriction imposed by the patient's condition or treatment. For example, the patient may be permitted unrestricted movement of the upper extremities but be restricted in the movement of one or both of the lower extremities. When possible, the patient should be encouraged to assist the nurse in changing his position by using self-help devices such as an overbed trapeze as shown in Fig. 2-6. The nurse assists the patient who is able to bear weight on the lower extremities to get out of bed and to stand by first moving the patient to a sitting position. The first step of getting the ambulatory patient

sitting

out of bed is to move him to a _____ position.

28 The nurse helps the patient from the sitting position to a standing position by lifting and pulling him as needed. In preparation for lifting and pulling the patient the nurse must:

a. Face the patient.

a. _____

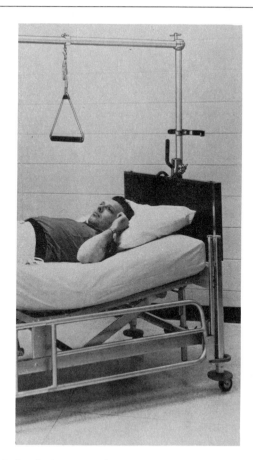

Fig. 2-6. Overbed trapeze. (Courtesy Zimmer · USA, Warsaw, Ind.)

17

b. Stand close to him.
c. Flex the knees.
d. Hold the back straight.
e. Contract muscles.

b. _____

c. _____

d. _____

e. _____

29 Unless his medical condition contraindicates it, the patient's posture should be like that of the nurse when he stands. The nurse should check these points of the patient's posture: _____,

head

chest; back; feet; abdomen

_____ , _____ , _____ , and _____ .
Note: the patient is able to walk or stand more easily in supportive shoes than in soft slippers or bare feet.

30 What would you check on each point mentioned in Frame 29?

a. Head is held up, chin in.
b. Chest is held so that the sternum is in front of the body.
c. Back is straight.
d. Abdomen is flat.
e. Feet are slightly apart and pointed straight ahead.

a. _____

b. _____

c. _____

d. _____

e. _____

31 Bedboards can be used under a mattress to create a firm surface that will be more comfortable and less fatiguing for the bed patient. The supine position is similar to the standing one, with minor variations such as a pillow being used to support the lumbar curve and

like

head. The supine position is (like? unlike?) the standing position.

32 To maintain normal functioning of the lungs, the head pillow should also be under the shoulders to allow complete expansion of the chest. To obtain a firm surface that is more comfortable and less

bedboards

fatiguing, _____ can be used.

To allow complete expansion of the chest or to permit normal functioning of the lungs.

33 Why should the head pillow also be placed under the shoulders?

34 All patients are predisposed to the development of deformities because of limited activity and the debilitating effects of disease. Preventable contractures and decubiti can be more serious, costly, and difficult to treat than the patient's original condition. To prevent them, the nurse must position the patient correctly, provide active or passive range of motion exercises, and change the patient's position frequently. Preventive measures that the nurse can control

correct position; exercises

change; position

are c_____ p_____ , e_____ , and frequent c_____ of p_____ .

35 The supine patient cannot maintain correct lower extremity position without assistance. After a short time, the anterior leg

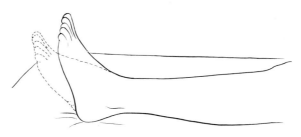

Fig. 2-7. Plantar flexion of the foot is illustrated by the broken line.

muscles are stretched and the foot assumes a plantar flexion position. A board or sandbag placed against the soles will prevent ''foot drop.'' Plantar flexion in time results in the contracture deformity known as _____ .

foot drop

36 Foot drop can be prevented by the use of _____ or _____ .

sandbags
foot boards

37 Relaxation of the muscles also allows external rotation of the legs. The nurse should place a sandbag against the bed patient's knee or thigh to maintain a proper relaxed position and to prevent _____ .

external rotation

38 Two deformities of the supine position that the nurse can prevent are: _____ and _____ _____ .

foot drop; external
rotation of the legs

39 Various devices are used to prevent deformities and to promote relaxation of the muscles. These include _____ and _____ .

foot boards
sandbags

40 When the patient is positioned on his side, the uppermost leg rests on the other leg, creating pressure areas and placing the leg in an adducted, internally rotated position. To keep this from occurring, the nurse supports the upper leg on a pillow. A pillow between the legs will retard development of _____ and keep the leg from assuming an _____ , _____ _____ position.

pressure areas
adducted; internally rotated

41 While in either the supine or side-lying position, the bed patient naturally holds his arms close to his body (adducted). Over a prolonged period of time, what may develop from the arms being held in the same position? _____

contractures

42 To maintain a functional position and to prevent contractures, the patient's arm must be held away from his body. This can be done

any supportive device

by using _____
between the body and the arm.

43 What preventable deformities or contractures commonly occur?

a. Foot drop
b. Internal and external rotation of the legs
c. Adducted arms

a. _____
b. _____
c. _____

44 Rehabilitation can be facilitated by the maintenance of function at the highest possible level during illness. The functions of the fingers and hands are essential and deserve more attention than they are usually allotted. The most essential function is the ability to pinch or grasp by touching the fingers with the thumb, as shown in Fig. 2-8. Sponge rubber rolls, rubber balls, rolled-up washcloths, and other devices should be used continuously to preserve this basic function. Why is maintenance of function of the fingers and hands so important?

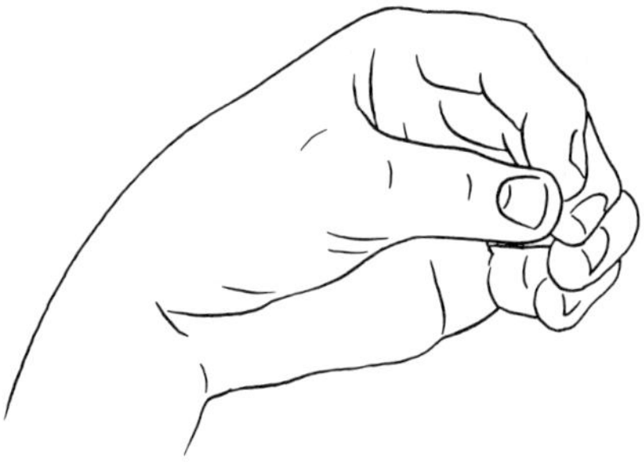

Because the ability to pinch or grasp is essential.

Fig. 2-8. Approximation of thumb and finger in the basic pinch or grasp position.

45 Maintenance of function should be extended particularly to the

fingers; hand

_____ and _____ .

Ability to grasp or pinch.

46 What is the most essential function of the hand?

47 List several devices that will help to preserve the functions of the hand.

a. Sponge rubber rolls
b. Rubber balls
c. Rolled-up washcloths

a. _____
b. _____
c. _____

20

48 In addition to being used to maintain a position, each of the devices can be utilized in a planned program of active or passive exercises. The patient can be encouraged to continue normal activities within his limitations as a part of the exercise program. Try to think of maintenance of function not as a haphazard thing but as part of a

planned   _____ program.

49 Muscle fatigue, strain, or spasm is often the source of discomfort for the orthopedic patient. A change of position, exercise, or additional support may bring relief without the use of medications. Some causes of discomfort for the orthopedic patient are:

muscle fatigue; strain   _____ , _____ ,

spasm   or _____ .

50 Within the limitations of the physician's instructions, the nurse should alter the patient's position. The prone position is rarely used, but it can be very restful for the bed patient. The nurse may relieve

changing his position; as-   the patient's discomfort by _____ ,
sisting him with exercises;   _____ , or
giving his body additional
support   _____ .

51 The prone position is most comfortable if one pillow is placed under the shoulders and chest, with another used beneath the feet and lower legs to keep the toes off the bed. The prone position is the reverse of the supine position, with pillows used under the

chest; shoulders; lower legs   _____ , _____ , _____ ,

feet   and _____ .

52 When the patient is moved, his joints must be supported to avoid muscle spasms or strain. When positioning a limb, the nurse should

joint   place a hand under the _____ to splint it.

53 Why does the nurse support the patient's joints when moving

To prevent muscle spasms,   him?
strain, or pain.

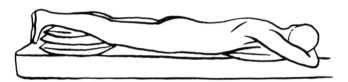

Fig. 2-9. Placement of pillows for comfort in the prone position.

21

54 Additional support that will make the patient more comfortable can be provided by strategically placed pillows or sandbags. In the side-lying position, the patient's back muscles can be supported by a pillow placed firmly against the back. Discomfort resulting from muscle fatigue may be eased by using _____ to _____ the affected areas.

55 Unless contraindicated, the nurse may elevate the patient's arm or leg. A changed position will be more comfortable if adequate support is provided for the limb during the move and afterward. The nurse supports the limb when moving it by _____ _____ .

56 Which portion of Fig. 2-10 represents the proper way to support an elevated leg? Why?

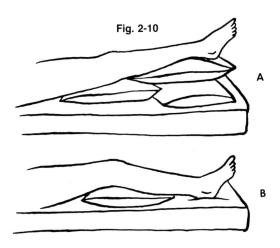

Fig. 2-10

57 Several days ago Mrs. Jones had surgery on her right knee. She has just asked for a pill to ease the pain. You could give her a pill, but you could also ease the pain by _____ _____ , _____ _____ , or _____ _____ .

58 Fig. 2-11 shows Mrs. Jones sitting in a chair. Which points of her posture need to be corrected?

22

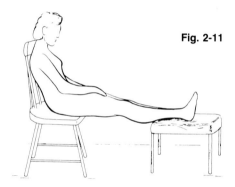

Fig. 2-11

59 Another nurse is going to assist you in lifting Mrs. Jones into bed since she is unable to stand. How would the two of you prepare yourselves to lift her?

a. Face her.
b. Stand close to her.
c. Keep back straight.
d. Flex your knees.
e. Contract muscles.

a. _____
b. _____
c. _____
d. _____
e. _____

60 You have decided to position Mrs. Jones on her left side. You would support her body by placing pillows _____

between her legs; between her right arm and her body; parallel with her back

_____ , _____ ,

and _____ .

61 The deformities that might have developed if she had not been

adducted, internally rotated right leg; adducted right arm

supported in this manner are _____

_____ and _____

_____ .

62 Later, Mrs. Jones complains of right knee pain and asks to be turned. Since dinner will be served soon, a supine or semi-Fowler's

easier

position would make it (easier? harder?) to change her to a sitting position.

63 The importance of the sitting position for meals is to (make the

allow the body to function normally

patient look and feel better? allow the body to function normally?).

64 While Mrs. Jones is in the supine position, you might reposition

elevated
relieve her pain

her right leg so it is _____ . This would help to

_____ .

65 In the supine position, Mrs. Jones might develop deformities

foot drop; external rotation of the legs

such as _____ or _____

_____ .

23

66 How can these deformities be prevented?

a. Foot drop—a foot board may be placed against the soles of the feet.
b. External rotation of the legs—sandbags can be placed against the knees and thighs.

a. _____
_____
_____

b. _____
_____
_____

67 The next morning Mrs. Jones is allowed to stand at the side of the bed. Since she looks like the person in Fig. 2-12, you would tell her to:

erect; chin
a. Hold her head _____ with her _____ in.

sternum; front
b. Hold her chest so her _____ is in _____ of the rest of her body.

straight
c. Hold her back _____ .

flat
d. Keep her abdomen _____ .

closer together
e. Place her feet _____ .

straight ahead
f. Point her feet _____ .

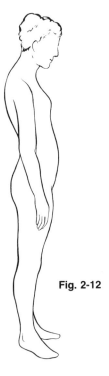

Fig. 2-12

68 Your knowledge of the principles of body mechanics will help you to _____

prevent injury to yourself; set a good example for your patients

and to _____ .

69 Application of body mechanics principles contributes to the attainment of nursing care goals. Which of the following nursing care goals would be influenced by application of body mechanics principles?

a, b, and d

a. Prevent hypostatic pneumonia
b. Maintain right leg in abducted, externally rotated position
c. Increase social interaction
d. Stimulate peristalsis

70 The principles of the functions of the muscles and joints are called _____ .

body mechanics

CHAPTER 3

Classification of fractures

■ Fractures are discussed as a separate orthopedic entity because they occur so frequently and patients with them are cared for in a variety of clinical settings. The hospital emergency department nurse, the hospital orthopedic unit nurse, the nurse in the physician's office, the public health nurse, and the primary nurse practitioner must be able to understand the terminology used to describe fractures and must understand the processes that occur at the time the bone is fractured. This chapter presents a brief discussion of the injuries associated with a fracture, the terms used to describe the anatomical location of a fracture, the terms used to describe the geometric patterns in which fractures occur, and other terms used in relation to fractures.

Fractures are classified according to several different attributes. The first classification is made on the basis of the nature of the wound, the second is made according to the part of the bone involved, while the third categorization is based on the general appearance or pattern of the fragments. Classic and descriptive names are also used to label fractures. The first three classifications are presented in this chapter. The classic and descriptive names require more in-depth study and the student-user is referred to the suggested readings at the end of the book.

B; break

1 Which part of Fig. 3-1 demonstrates continuity of the bone? _____ A fracture is a _____ in the continuity of a bone.

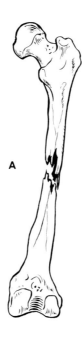

Fig. 3-1

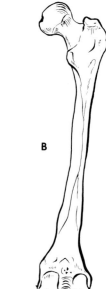

A

B

2 The layman thinks of a fracture as just a broken bone, but tissues, blood vessels, and periosteum are also involved. At the time of fracture, the soft tissues and blood vessels are injured and the periosteum is torn away from the bone (Fig. 3-2). When a bone is fractured, s_____ t_____ and b_____ v_____ are damaged, and the p_____ is stripped away from the bone.

soft tissues; blood vessels; periosteum

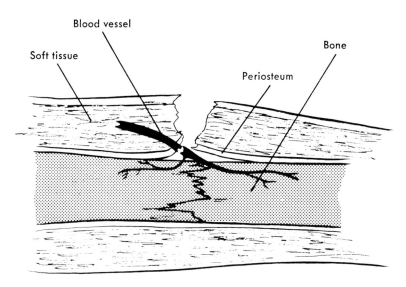

Fig. 3-2

3 Further injury may occur from the movements of the pieces of bone. The bone pieces are fragments. Ultimate cure depends upon restoration of the bony fragments, _____, _____, and _____.

soft tissues
blood vessels; periosteum

4 Label Fig. 3-3 correctly.

A. _____
B. _____
C. _____
D. _____

A. Periosteum
B. Blood vessel
C. Soft tissue
D. Bone fragment

5 Fractures are characterized by the presence of swelling and hemorrhage. The swelling and hemorrhage are the result of injury to the _____ and _____.

blood vessels; soft tissue

6 The bone fragments are labeled as being either *distal* or *proximal,* according to their relationship to the center of the body. Distal suggests distance or away from. Proximal, therefore, very likely means (near to? far from?) the center of the body.

near to

27

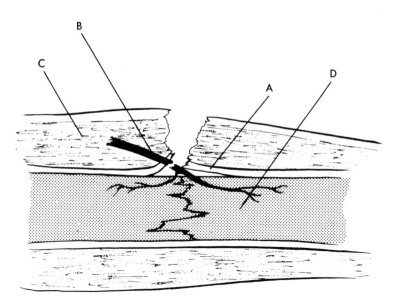

Fig. 3-3

proximal

7 The fragment nearest the center of the body is the (proximal? distal?) fragment.

8 Label the distal and proximal fragments in Fig. 3-4.

A. Proximal
B. Distal

A. _____

B. _____

9 The first classification of fractures is determined by whether the wound is *open* or *closed*. In an open fracture, the bone has penetrated the skin and the wound is open to external contamination. In a closed fracture, you could expect that the bone (has? has not?) penetrated the skin. Label the open and closed fractures in Fig. 3-5.

has not

A. Closed
B. Open

A. _____

B. _____

10 How is a fracture classified when the skin is penetrated by a bone fragment? _____

open

11 In a closed fracture, the bone (does? does not?) come through the skin.

does not

12 What complication is likely to result from an open fracture? _____

infection

13 Define open and closed fractures.

Open—bone fragment penetrates the skin. Closed—bone fragment does not penetrate the skin.

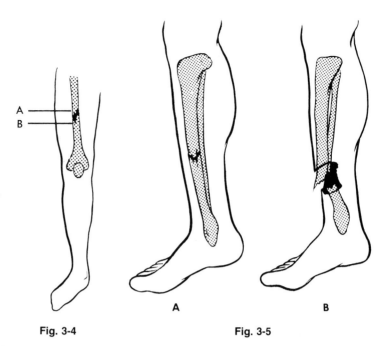

Fig. 3-4

Fig. 3-5

14 The second classification of fractures describes the portion of the bone which has been fractured. Use of this classification requires the utilization of anatomical terms with which the reader should be familiar. Match the anatomical description (left column) with the appropriate phrase (right column).

b

c

a

_____ 1. Articular   a. Within a joint cavity

_____ 2. Periarticular   b. Involving joint surface

_____ 3. Intra-articular   c. Near to but not involving a joint

15 In addition to the previous terms, the labels intra- and extra-capsular may be utilized to describe the location of the fracture in relation to a joint. Since intracapsular refers to a fracture within the joint capsule, fractures near to but outside of the joint capsular would

extracapsular

be _____ .

16 The term extracapsular provides a description very much like the

peri

term _____articular.

17 The term intracapsular does not provide a description of the location of the fracture as specific as the terms _____

articular

intra-articular

and _____ .

18 The long bones, especially the humerus and femur, can be divided into four basic sections, as shown in Fig. 3-6. An apophyseal fracture is typically an avulsion fracture of an apophysis where there

is not

is a strong tendinous attachment. The apophysis (is? is not?) a part of the joint.

19 Referring to Fig. 3-6, the long shaft of the bone is the

diaphysis

_____ .

20 The epiphysis of the bone is the end of the bone and is usually wider than the shaft and is separated from the shaft by a cartilaginous disk. The epiphysis may also be fractured, which would then be a fracture within the joint. The following terms could be used to de-

intracapsular

articular; intra-articular

scribe an epiphyseal fracture: _____ ,

_____ ,

and/or _____ .

21 The metaphysis is the portion of a long bone between the shaft and the wide parts of the ends. If the femoral metaphysis at the end of the femur closer to the knee were fractured, the fracture could

distal

be labeled as a (proximal? distal?) metaphyseal fracture.

22 A fracture of the shaft of the bone may also be referred to as a

diaphysis

fracture of the _____ .

23 An avulsion fracture where the tendinous attachment of the bone

apophyseal

is torn away is a(n) _____ fracture.

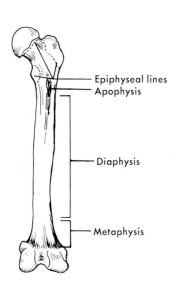

Epiphyseal lines
Apophysis

Diaphysis

Metaphysis

Fig. 3-6. Anatomic structure of long bone.

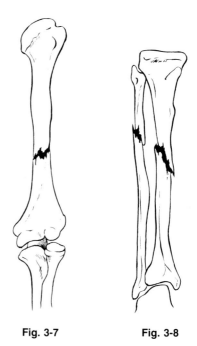

Fig. 3-7   Fig. 3-8

Fig. 3-7. Transverse fracture of the humerus.
Fig. 3-8. Oblique fracture of the fibula and tibia.

a. Apophysis
b. Diaphysis
c. Metaphysis
d. Epiphysis

shapes
patterns

transverse

right
does not

A. Oblique
B. Transverse

oblique
sharper; climbing

24 The four major anatomical locations on a long bone are:

a. _____

b. _____

c. _____

d. _____

25 The third classification of fractures is based on the *shape* or *pattern* of the fracture. Fractures occur in basic _____ or _____ .

26 The transverse fracture is characterized by the fracture line forming a right angle with the shaft of the bone and is most common in the long bones. The fracture that forms a right angle with the shaft of the bone is the _____ .

27 The oblique fracture line slants at an angle across the shaft of the bone. The transverse fracture line forms a _____ angle with the shaft of the bone and the oblique (does? does not?).

28 Classify each fracture in Fig. 3-9 according to pattern.

A. _____

B. _____

29 The spiral pattern is usually the result of twisting action such as occurs in a skiing accident. The pattern is similar to the oblique in angle, but the angle is sharper and appears to be climbing. The spiral fracture is like the _____ but somewhat different in that it is _____ and _____ .

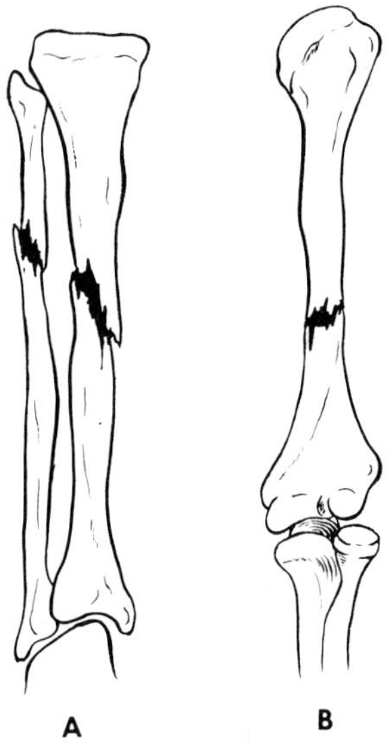

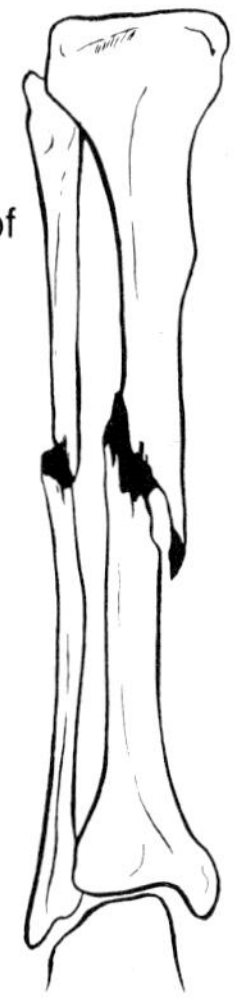

Fig. 3-10. Spiral fracture of the fibula and tibia.

A   B

Fig. 3-9

30 A sharp angle and a climbing appearance are characteristic of the _____ fracture.

spiral

31 A twisting action usually results in a _____ fracture.

spiral

32 The three fracture patterns that form an angle with the shaft of the bones are: _____ , _____ , and _____ .

oblique; transverse
spiral

33 The fracture line of the comminuted fracture does not form a well-defined, specific angle with the shaft of the bone. Fig. 3-11 shows a broken bone where the fracture line does not intersect the bone shaft at a specific angle. The figure shows a _____ fracture.

comminuted

34 In addition to the fact that a comminuted fracture (does? does not?) form an angle, a comminuted fracture is also characterized by the presence of more than two fragments. Which portion of Fig. 3-12 shows a comminuted fracture? _____ How many fragments does it show? _____

does not

B

four

35 In Fig. 3-12, *B*, the smaller fragments appear to be (attached to? floating between?) the larger fragments.

floating between

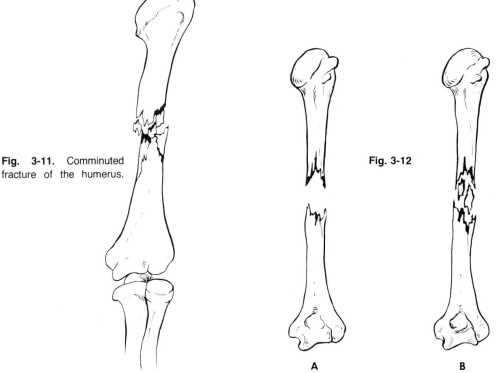

Fig. 3-11. Comminuted fracture of the humerus.

Fig. 3-12

A   B

32

36 In the comminuted fracture there are _____ _____ fragments and they appear to be _____ between the proximal and distal fragments.

more than two

floating

37 What are the characteristics of the comminuted fracture?

a. _____
_____

b. _____
_____

c. _____
_____

a. There are more than two fragments.
b. The fracture line does not form an angle with the shaft of the bone.
c. The small fragments appear to be floating between the larger fragments.

38 At other times, the fragments of a comminuted fracture of a large bone may be forced together or impacted rather than floating freely between the other fragments of the bone. In an impacted fracture the fragments are (free floating? forced together?).

forced together

39 The compression fracture is similar to the comminuted, impacted fracture in that there are more than two fragments that are forced together. However, the term compression fracture is used to describe the appearance of small bones, usually the vertebrae. Which part of Fig. 3-13 demonstrates a compression fracture? _____ Which part demonstrates a comminuted fracture? _____

B

C

(A shows the normal size and shape of a vertebra.)

Fig. 3-13

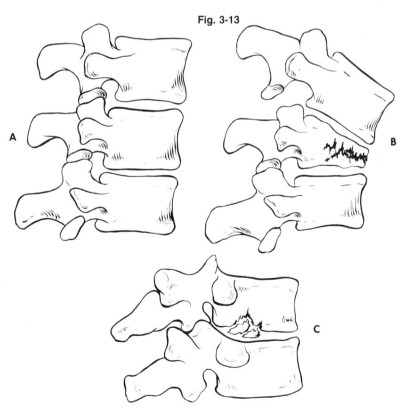

A

B

C

33

40 In the compression fracture, the bone appears to be (smaller? normal?) in size.

41 The compression fracture is (like? unlike?) the comminuted fracture because there are (only two? more than two?) bone fragments present.

42 In both the compression and comminuted fractures, the fracture line (does? does not?) form an angle with the shaft of the bone.

43 What are the characteristics of the compression fracture?

a. _____
_____

b. _____
_____

c. _____
_____

44 How is the compression fracture similar to the comminuted fracture?

45 The equivalent of a compression fracture involving a long bone is a(n) _____ fracture.

46 The greenstick fracture is an incomplete fracture open on only one side of the bone. It splits longitudinally. Only children sustain

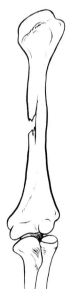

Fig. 3-14. Greenstick fracture of the humerus.

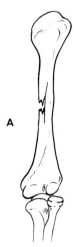

A

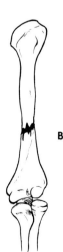

B

Fig. 3-15

greenstick fractures. The fracture line of a greenstick fracture is (longitudinal? at an angle?) and (complete? incomplete?).

longitudinal; incomplete

47 An incomplete fracture open on only one side and with a longitudinal split is a(n) _____ fracture.

greenstick

48 What fracture is incurred only by children? _____

greenstick

49 Adults may also sustain fractures that do not result in any one of the preceding patterns because the fracture is incomplete. A longitudinal fracture that runs parallel to the length of a long bone may be incurred. A longitudinal fracture is incomplete because at the time of fracture the periosteum is not _____ _____ .

torn away from the bone

50 The two types of incomplete fractures are the _____ and the _____ .

longitudinal
greenstick

51 Correctly label the fractures in Fig. 3-15.
A. _____
B. _____

A. Greenstick
B. Transverse

52 Label each of the drawings in Fig. 3-16 with the correct fracture pattern name.
A. _____
B. _____
C. _____
D. _____
E. _____
F. _____

A. Oblique
B. Spiral
C. Compression
D. Comminuted
E. Greenstick
F. Transverse

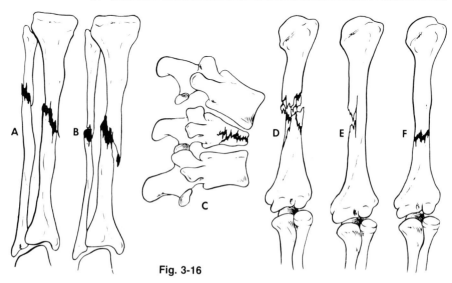

Fig. 3-16

53 What are the characteristics of the comminuted fracture?

a. It has more than two fragments.
b. The smaller fragments appear to be floating.
c. The fracture line does not form a definite angle with the bone shaft.

a. _____
_____

b. _____
_____

c. _____
_____

54 How is the compression fracture different from the comminuted fracture?

The fragments are pushed together and the bone seems smaller in the compression fracture.

55 What are the characteristics of the spiral fracture?

a. It has a sharp angle.
b. It has a climbing appearance.

a. _____

b. _____

56 In what pattern does the fracture line form a right angle with the bone shaft? _____

transverse

57 Other than by pattern, how may a fracture be described?

a. Open or closed
b. Anatomical site

a. _____

b. _____

58 What is an open fracture?

An open fracture is one in which the bone fragments penetrate the skin.

59 Define fracture.

A fracture is an interruption in the continuity of a bone.

60 Healing depends upon restoration of the _____

bone fragments; soft tissues; blood vessels; periosteum

_____ , _____ , _____
_____ , and _____ .

36

CHAPTER 4

Stages of bone healing

1 The healing process in a bone occurs in stages and is referred to as *union*. The injuries occurring at the time of fracture are to the

periosteum; soft tissues
blood vessels
union

bone, _____, _____, and _____. The healing process is (reconstruction? union? restoration?).

2 The length of time required to complete the healing process depends upon the age of the patient and the size of the fractured bone. The rate of union in influenced by what two factors?

a. Age of patient
b. Size of the fractured bone

a. _____
b. _____

3 The younger patient usually heals more rapidly than the older patient, and smaller bones usually heal more rapidly than larger (long) bones. Union will occur more slowly when:

a. The patient is older
b. A large (long) bone is fractured

a. _____
b. _____

4 The first stage of union is the formation of a blood clot or hematoma that surrounds the damaged structures. *Hematoma formation* is the first stage of bone healing. Swelling and hemorrhage are two

hematoma

signs of a fracture, and they precede _____ formation.

A blood clot forms around the damaged structures.

5 Describe the first stage of bone healing.

6 A few days after the fracture occurs, the hematoma changes with the invasion of granulation tissue. *Granulation* is the second stage

hematoma formation
granulation

of union. The first stage of union is (hemorrhage? hematoma formation? swelling?). The second stage of union is _____.

7 The granulation tissue contains blood vessels, fibroblasts, and osteoblasts, which produce a substance called *osteoid*. As minerals are deposited in the osteoid in the following weeks, *callus formation*

By minerals being deposited in the osteoid.

occurs. How is a callus formed?

37

8 List the stages of union to this point.

a. _____

b. _____

c. _____

9 As the osteoblasts and fibroblasts continue to multiply, the distance between the fragments is closed and *consolidation* or *ossification* takes place. What occurs during consolidation?

10 When consolidation is completed, the excess cells are absorbed, the bone is *remodeled,* and union is complete. Number the stages of union listed below in the order of their occurrence.

_____ Consolidation

_____ Callus formation

_____ Remodeling

_____ Granulation

_____ Hematoma formation

11 Briefly describe each stage of union.

a. Hematoma formation _____

_____

b. Granulation _____

_____

c. Callus formation _____

_____

d. Consolidation (ossification) _____

_____

e. Remodeling _____

_____

12 Patient A is 6 years old and has a fractured clavicle. Patient B is 40 years old and has a fractured clavicle. In which patient would union generally occur first? Why?

13 Patient A is 40 years old and has a fractured femur. Patient B is 40 years old and has a fractured calcaneus. In which patient would union usually occur first? Why?

14 The osteoid is produced by (periosteum? fibroblasts? osteocytes? osteoblasts?).

15 List the stages of union.

a. Hematoma formation   a. _____

b. Granulation   b. _____

c. Callus formation   c. _____

d. Consolidation   d. _____

e. Remodeling   e. _____

CHAPTER 5

Complications of fractures

■ The nursing care of the patient who has a fracture should be focused on the prevention of complications and the early recognition of signs and symptoms of associated complications and injuries and fat embolism. The nursing care of the patient whose complications are directly related to the fracture itself is based on the treatment prescribed by the physician.

prevention

1 One of the complications directly related to the fracture itself is a bone *infection,* which is extremely serious; it is discussed in Chapter 16. Bone infections can be prevented by the proper first aid and emergency care of an open fracture and by strict observance of aseptic technique during an open reduction. Nursing care of the fracture patient should be focused on the _____ of infection.

proper first aid and emergency care of an open fracture; strict observance of aseptic technique during an open reduction

2 Bone infections can be prevented by _____ _____ and by _____ _____ .

infection

nonunion

3 *Nonunion* of a bone is failure of the bone fragments to grow together, with changes that indicate a permanent state. Two complications related to the fracture itself are _____ and _____ .

permanent

4 Nonunion is accompanied by indications that it is a (temporary? permanent?) state.

are not

5 Delayed union is retarded healing beyond the normal rate. Delayed union and nonunion (are? are not?) the same.

crooked

6 Malunion is union of the fragments in a deformed position. If the patient has malunion of his fractured femur, you would reason that his femur is (straight? crooked?).

longer than usual

7 If the same patient also has delayed union, his fracture healed in a (normal? longer than usual?) amount of time.

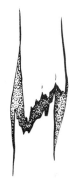

Fig. 5-1. Malunion of fracture fragments.

infection; nonunion

malunion; delayed union

8 The complications of fractures directly related to the fracture itself are _____ , _____ , _____ , and _____ .

death

9 *Avascular necrosis* is death of a bone from deficient blood supply. The term *necrosis* is associated with the word _____ .

it has a poor blood supply

10 In avascular necrosis, the bone dies because (it has been broken? it has a poor blood supply?).

different from

11 Avascular necrosis is (the same as? different from?) nonunion.

different from

12 Avascular necrosis is (the same as? different from?) delayed union.

13 The psychologic care of the patient whose fracture is complicated must take into consideration the length of time the patient has been incapacitated or hospitalized and the effect this has on him. Two patients the same age were injured on the same day. They both sustained closed fractures of the tibia that were treated in essentially the same manner. The first patient's fracture has healed, the second patient's fracture has not. What complications related to the fracture itself might the second patient have?

a. Nonunion
b. Delayed union
c. Avascular necrosis
   (Since they were closed fractures, infection was less likely as a complication.)

a. _____
b. _____
c. _____

14 The physical care of the patient whose fracture is complicated by infection, malunion, nonunion, delayed union, or avascular necrosis is based on the treatment modality selected by the physician. Unfortunately, fractures are sometimes complicated by concomitant injuries or physiologically related consequences of a fracture. Nursing care of the fracture patient should include measures designed to prevent physiologically related consequences such as compartment syndrome and fat embolism. At the same time the nurse must observe the patient for signs and symptoms of fat emboli and compartment syndrome since preventive efforts may not always be successful.

15 Compartment syndrome is a complication that may be indirectly related to the fracture and/or the mode of treatment of an otherwise uncomplicated fracture. That is, compartment syndrome may occur spontaneously or as a result of the therapy modality. For example, compartment syndrome may develop after a plaster cast has been applied to the fractured limb. Compartment syndrome is a complication related to the method of treating a fracture. (Never? Sometimes? Always?)

Sometimes

16 Groups of muscles in the extremities are enclosed in a sheath of fascia with narrow entry and exit ports at each end for nerves and blood vessels. The fascia sheath surrounds the muscles, nerves, and blood vessels to form a _____.

compartment
(You may need to review the anatomy of the musculo-skeletal system.)

17 Compartment syndrome is a progressive vascular compromise of a portion of an extremity which, if untreated, can result in permanent injury of the muscles and nerves within the involved compartment. Compartment syndrome is basically a _____ problem.

vascular

18 Vascular compromise is part of a vicious circle of phenomena. The compromise or blocking of the blood supply is the result of trauma to the muscle, which results in edema. The muscular trauma may stem from a fracture or a cast or bandage. When a muscle has a decreased flow of oxygenated blood, it is _____.

ischemic

19 Trauma leads to edema, and edema leads to ischemia. Ischemia then leads to additional edema since the muscle's response to ischemia is to release histamine, which causes capillary dilation that is followed by the transudation of plasma into the muscle and thereby produces additional muscular edema. The ischemia-edema-ischemia circle takes place within the muscle compartment, which is nonexpanding. Since the fascia does not expand with the increased edema, the pressure against the contents of the compartment (increases? decreases?).

increases

20 As the pressure within the compartment increases, the blood vessels are further occluded, which again leads to ischemia that in turn causes compression of the small veins and arteries within the muscle substance, leading to occlusion of large arteries and further reduction of blood flow. The vicious circle of vascular compromise can be described as (regression? degenerative? excessive? progressive?).

progressive

21 As the vascular compromise within the compartment progresses, the occlusion leads to further muscle edema. As the swelling increases, the nerve traversing the compartment becomes ischemic and nerve function is lost. This chain of events may have been triggered by:

All of these

a. A fracture fragment pressing on an artery
b. A cast that was too tight and blocked the blood supply
c. A bandage that was too tight and blocked the flow of blood
d. Any tissue trauma that leads to swelling within the compartment

22 Continued compression of the blood vessels leads to loss of muscle function from tissue anoxia and eventually tissue infarction. Irreversible tissue damage will occur within the compartment unless the vicious circle of edema-ischemia is interrupted. Infarcted muscle will eventually develop into a contracture. Compartment syndrome must be prevented or recognized early in order to prevent permanent

nerve; muscle

_____ and _____ damage.

23 The muscle groups most commonly affected are those in the forearm and lower leg. A supracondylar fracture of the elbow and a fracture of the proximal tibia are the most commonly identified fractures associated with compartment syndrome. Compartment syn-

edema-ischemia

drome is described as a vicious circle of _____ .

24 Compartment syndrome may be prevented by measures being

edema
(The circle starts with edema.)

taken to prevent the development of _____ .

25 In future chapters, nursing measures that can be taken to prevent the development of edema after a fracture will be discussed. The discussion will not be limited to prevention of compartment syndrome specifically but will refer to prevention of complications generally. Although preventive measures may have been instituted, the nurse remains responsible for observation of the patient for indications of fracture complications.

26 The signs and symptoms of compartment syndrome are indicative of the degree of involvement or progression of damage. The earliest indication of compartment syndrome is progressive, abnormal pain. The fracture patient naturally will have some pain, but analgesics relieve normal fracture-related pain fairly readily. The pain associated with compartment syndrome is not relieved by analgesics; instead, it becomes progressively more intense and is general rather than being localized to the fracture site. The first indication

progressive abnormal pain
(Note that edema of the digits of the affected limb is not *an indication of compartment syndrome.)*

of compartment syndrome is _____

_____ .

27 Pain on passive movement of the digits is also an early indication of compartment syndrome. How does the pain associated with compartment syndrome differ from the pain usually associated with a fracture?

It is progressively more intense, is not relieved by analgesics, and occurs with passive movement of the digits.

28 Either paresthesia or paralysis may be observed next as the pressure within the compartment increases. Paresthesia and paralysis indicate that the involved nerve's sensory and motor functions have been affected. Loss of sensory function results in

paresthesia

_____, and loss of motor function results

paralysis

in _____ .

29 Mrs. Jones fractured her right ulna when she fell on the ice 3 hours ago. She now complains of numbness and tingling in her fingers. The nurse asked her to describe any pain she might have, to move her fingers, and to move her fingers passively. The nurse

paresthesia (numbness and tingling) is an indication of compartment syndrome

carried out these steps because _____

_____ .

30 Paresthesia and paralysis are relatively late signs of compart-

abnormal progressive pain; pain on passive movement of the digits

ment syndrome; the early signs are _____

_____ and _____

_____ .

31 Pallor of the digits and pulselessness distal to fracture site are such late signs of compartment syndrome that by the time they are noted permanent damage may have occurred. List the signs and symptoms of compartment syndrome in sequence according to their value as indications of compartment syndrome.

a. Abnormal, progressive pain
b. Pain on passive movement
c. Paresthesia
d. Paralysis
e. Pallor
f. Pulselessness

a. _____

b. _____

c. _____

d. _____

e. _____

f. _____

32 Compartment syndrome is treated by removal of any external constrictions from around the affected limb, including a cast and other immobilizing bandages, followed by elevation of the extremity to aid venous return. Casts and bandages may have prevented any possible compartment expansion as swelling occurred. The cast or bandage per se need not be removed but their constriction around the affected limb must be released. For example, a cast can be split

lengthwise and loosely taped in place. The initial treatment is to
ensure that the _____ is not constricted.

compartment

33 Since the swelling occurs within the compartment and the compartment can expand only a finite amount, the compartment must be opened if previous attempts at treatment are unsuccessful. Fasciotomy, as the term implies, means cutting into fascia; this surgical decompression procedure permits the swelling to continue unrestricted (without putting pressure on the blood vessels, nerves, and/or muscle). Surgical decompression of the compartment is achieved by _____ .

fasciotomy

34 The nurse should report the early indications of compartment syndrome so that treatment may be instituted immediately. The treatment of compartment syndrome includes _____
_____ , _____
_____ and _____ .

removing external constrictions; elevation of the extremity; fasciotomy

35 The complications indirectly related to fractures include fat embolism and injury to major blood vessels, nerves, viscera, and tendons. The nursing care of fracture patients, therefore, should be focused on the early recognition of the signs and symptoms of associated complications. The nurse needs to know the signs and symptoms of injury to the b_____ v_____ ,
v_____ , n_____ , and t_____ .

blood vessels

viscera; nerves; tendons

36 Many of the signs and symptoms of fracture-related complications overlap; that is, one sign or symptom may be indicative of more than one kind of injury. The nurse does not determine which injury has occurred but immediately reports observation to the physician. Some of the signs and symptoms that may be indicative of injury to blood vessels, nerves, viscera, or tendons are changes in the size (swelling), skin temperature, color, or appearance of the affected extremity; changes in the function or motion of the affected extremity; abnormal or decreased sensations of the affected extremity; and signs of hemorrhage including increased drainage or bleeding. Indicate which complications are (a) *directly* related to the fracture, and (b) *indirectly* related to the fracture.

b   _____ Ruptured spleen

b   _____ Severed artery

a   _____ Delayed union

a   _____ Avascular necrosis

b   _____ Severed nerve

a   _____ Bone infection

b   _____ Pulmonary embolism

a   _____ Malunion

b   _____ Compartment syndrome

37 On arrival in the emergency room, the patient is complaining of pain and tingling in his fractured arm. The nurse notes that the patient's fingers are cool and slightly cyanotic. Should the nurse report these signs and symptoms? Why?

Yes; They may be indicative of injury to the blood vessels, nerves, or tendons or of compartment syndrome.

38 At the time of fracture, fat cells within the marrow of the bone may enter the bloodstream. The exact mechanism by which this process occurs is unknown. The fat globules are transported, via the circulatory system, to the lungs and cause a hemorrhagic interstitial pneumonitis that frequently leads to adult respiratory distress syndrome. One of the most serious complications of a fracture is

fat embolism

——————————————— .

39 Early recognition and treatment of fat embolism are essential since untreated emobli may be fatal in a very short period of time. Symptoms ˙of fat embolism may appear within 12 to 72 hours after the fracture. Fat embolism is characterized by changes in the patient's mental state, neurological signs, respiratory function, cardiac function, and body temperature. Most of these changes can be related to the resultant hypoxia. The signs for which the nurse should observe the fracture patient include:

a, c, d, e, f, h, and i

a. Tachypnea   f. Delirium
b. Hypoglycemia   g. Dementia
c. Confusion   h. Apprehension
d. Cyanosis   i. Tachycardia
e. Dyspnea

40 In addition, petechial hemorrhages appear on the anterior upper trunk, neck, head, conjunctiva, and soft palate. The mechanism of petechial hemorrhage is not well understood; however, the changes in the patient's mental state and neurological signs can be attributed

hypoxia

to ——————————— .

41 The patient's chest x-ray will reveal "snowstorm" pulmonary infiltrates or multiple areas of consolidation. Blood gas laboratory values will change as is consistent with adult respiratory distress syndrome. These findings imply that the treatment should include the administration of oxygen. It may be necessary to intubate the patient and place him on a respirator in order to provide the needed

oxygen

oxygen. The main problem in fat embolism is poor ——————————— exchange. The primary method of treatment is the administration of

oxygen

——————————— .

42 Additional treatment consists of the administration of corticosteroids and, at times, anticoagulants. Intravenous fluids are used to maintain nutrition and hydration. Which of the following laboratory test values must the orthopedic nurse be able to interpret?

a, c, and d

a. Serum electrolytes
b. Cholesterol esters
c. Arterial blood gases
d. Prothrombin time

43 When a patient has a fat embolism, the signs and symptoms include changes in _____ , _____

mental state; neurological signs; respiratory function; cardiac function; body temperature; chest x-ray and blood gas studies; skin appearance (petechiae)

_____ , _____

_____ , _____ ,

_____ , _____

_____ , and _____

_____ .

44 Select the states that occur as signs and symptoms of fat emboli.

a   ____ 1. Mental state   a. Confused   b. Alert
a   ____ 2. Neurological signs   a. Dilated pupils   b. Normal pupils
a, b   ____ 3. Respiratory functions   a. Dyspnea   b. Tachypnea
b   ____ 4. Cardiac function   a. Bradycardia   b. Tachycardia
b   ____ 5. Chest x-ray   a. Fluid present   b. "Snowstorm"
b   ____ 6. Blood gases   a. Elevated Pao_2 b. Decreased Pao_2
b   ____ 7. Skin appearance   a. Pallor   b. Petechiae

45 During the night the patient begins showing signs of a fat embolus. The patient, as occurs frequently, tells the nurse that he has a feeling of impending disaster or death, and in a short time his color changes from pale to _____ .

cyanotic

46 After treatment for the fat embolus, the patient progresses nicely and is discharged. Two months later he is readmitted for treatment of a complication. The complication, which necessitates further treatment, is directly related to the fracture. List the possible complications the patient might have.

a. Malunion
b. Nonunion
c. Delayed union
d. Avascular necrosis
e. Infection

a. _____
b. _____
c. _____
d. _____
e. _____

47 Sensations of pain, numbness, tingling or pressure, changes in the color, skin temperature, or function of the affected part, swelling, bleeding or drainage, and limited motion should be reported. These signs and symptoms may be indicative of injury to _____

blood vessels

nerves; viscera

tendons

_____ , _____ , _____ ,

or _____ .

48 A patient is admitted to the orthopedic unit with an open fracture of the distal third of the right femur. Select the observations made by the nurse that should be reported.

a, c, and d

a. Toes are cool and cyanotic
b. Has ingrown toenail on right foot
c. Right knee is edematous
d. Patient complaining of numbness in right foot
e. Dressing is dry

49 The reportable patient sensations, in addition to numbness, are

pain; tingling; pressure

_____ , _____ , and _____ .

50 The signs and symptoms of compartment syndrome include:

abnormal progressive pain;
pain on passive movement;
paresthesia; paralysis;
pallor; pulselessness

_____ ,
_____ ,
_____ , _____ ,
_____ , and _____ .

Delayed union and nonunion share the characteristic of a slower than normal rate of healing. Delayed union is unlike nonunion because healing will occur eventually, while in nonunion the changes indicate a permanent state.

51 Compare and contrast delayed union and nonunion.

Malunion is the union of the fragments in a deformed position.

52 Define malunion.

B

53 What portion of Fig. 5-2 demonstrates malunion? _____

Fig. 5-2

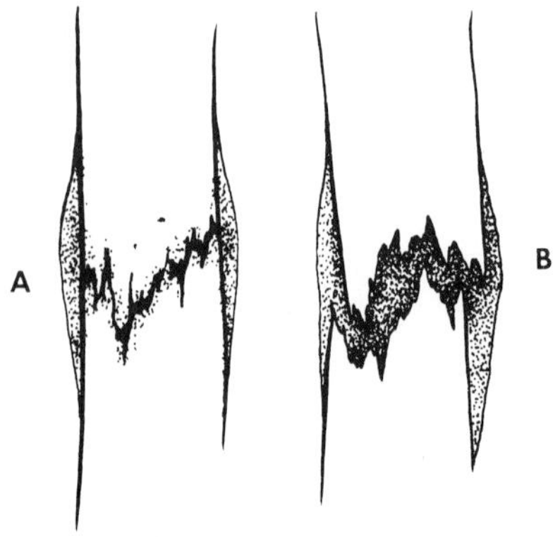

54 The nursing care of the patient who has a fracture should be focused on:

a. _____
_____

b. _____
_____

c. _____
_____

d. _____
_____

55 Which statements regarding fat emboli patients are true?

a. The onset of the emboli is at time of injury.
b. The mental confusion is due to low PCO_2.
c. Petechiae are the first sign of fat emobli.
d. Corticosteroid therapy is used as treatment.
e. Mechanical respirators may be used.
f. The patient may feel something is happening.

56 Multiple trauma victims present a challenge to the nurse because:

a. These are the sickest patients on the unit.
b. These patients must be observed closely for complications.
c. The nurse must integrate knowledge of medicine, surgery, and orthopedics in their care.
d. They tend to remain in the hospital a long time and can become tiresome to care for.

57 The three most serious complications of fractures are: _____
_____ , _____ , and _____ .

58 Complications directly related to the fracture are _____ ,
_____ , _____ , and
_____ .

59 The fracture patient with complications will experience some degree of psychological stress. The nurse can assist the patient in dealing with this stress by allowing the patient to freely verbalize his feelings, by guiding him in the selection of socially acceptable coping mechanisms, and by referring him to the appropriate persons or agency for additional assistance.

60 Discuss how the *Standards of Orthopedic Nursing Practice* (p. ix) are applicable to the care of the fracture patient with complications. Discuss your response with your instructor, classmates, or co-workers.

TREATMENT OF ORTHOPEDIC CONDITIONS

The medical and nursing treatment of orthopedic conditions is directed toward restoration of function to the affected part. Various methods or combinations of methods may be used by the physician to attain this goal. Some of the methods that may be utilized in the treatment of orthopedic conditions include surgical procedures that stabilize a bone or joint or correct a deformity (see Section Three), metallic fixation, traction, and cast immobilization. This section presents a description of these treatment modalities and the related nursing care.

CHAPTER 6

Treatment of fractures

1 After a bone is fractured, malunion may occur unless the fragments are realigned and held in position until union occurs. *Reduction* is the process of returning the fragments to their proper alignment and length. A broken bone appears to be (shorter? longer?) than a normal bone.

shorter

2 Certain fractures may be reduced by manipulating the fragments while the patient is anesthetized or sedated *(closed reduction)*. Define reduction.

Reduction is the process of returning the fragments to their proper alignment and length.

3 For other fractures, a surgical procedure *(open reduction)* may be necessary if traction or closed reduction are not appropriate. Manipulation of the fragments while the patient is sedated or anesthetized is a(n) _____ reduction.

closed

4 Surgical intervention to realign the fragments is (open? closed?) reduction.

open

5 Match the word with the appropriate definition.

c

_____ 1. Process of returning the fragments to their proper alignment

a. Open reduction

b. Closed reduction

a

_____ 2. Surgical intervention to realign the fragments

c. Reduction

b

_____ 3. Manipulation of the fragments while the patient is sedated or anesthetized.

6 *Traction* is the process of pulling either manually or by a system of ropes, pulleys, and weights. Traction may be used not only to reduce the fracture but also to maintain the reduction. The methods used by the physician to reduce a fracture are (closed reduction? manipulation? open reduction? traction?).

closed reduction, open reduction, traction

7 Prevention of movement of the fragments is *immobilization*. Immobilization maintains the desired alignment of the fragments while

53

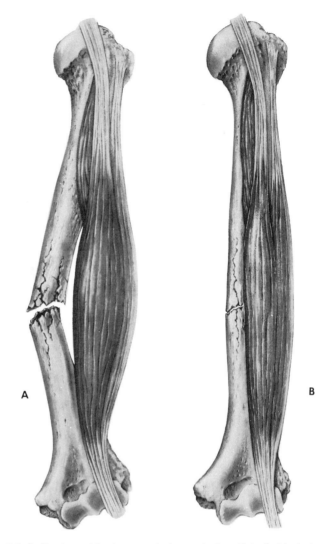

Fig. 6-1. A, Fracture of the humerus before reduction. Note that by being out of alignment the bone appears to be shorter. **B,** Fracture of the humerus after reduction. The fragments are realigned and the length of the bone has been restored. (Courtesy Zimmer · USA, Warsaw, Ind.)

union occurs. A fracture can be immobilized by using (open reduc-
traction   tion? traction? closed reduction?).

Fractures are reduced and   **8** Briefly describe how fractures are treated.
immobilized.

9 When an open reduction is performed, the physician may utilize metallic devices to hold the fragments in alignment. The use of pins, screws, nails, and plates to immobilize a fracture is *metallic fixation*.
prevention of movement of   Immobilization is the (prevention of movement of the fragments?
the fragments   retention of the fragments?).

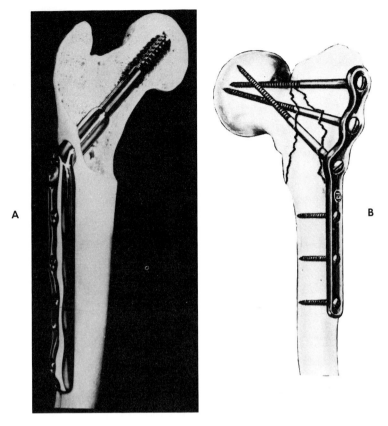

Fig. 6-2. A, Richards hip nail. (Courtesy Richards Mfg. Co., Memphis.) **B,** Moe bone plate held in place by bone screws immobilizes the fracture fragments. (Courtesy Zimmer · USA, Warsaw, Ind.)

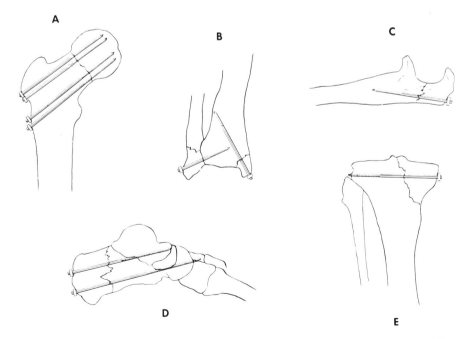

Fig. 6-3. Metallic fixation with one or more Knowles pins used to immobilize fracture fragments. The Knowles pin, as shown, can be used for fractures in numerous anatomic locations. (Courtesy Richards Mfg. Co., Memphis.)

10 The physician may insert a pin or nail directly into the medullary canal of the bone. After an intramedullary pin is inserted, the physician may slip a circumferential partial contact band around the fracture site. The band holds the fragments in place and yet minimizes the tendency for the bone to necrotize. The use of an intramedullary pin or nail to immobilize the fragments would be one form of open reduction with ______________________.

metallic fixation

11 Compression plating is another form of metallic fixation utilized to immobilze fracture fragments. Compression plating may also be thought of as a means of reducing the fracture since the fragment alignment is changed somewhat as the compression is applied. That is, the bone fragments are compressed into alignment by means of a compression device, as shown in Fig. 6-5, *B*. Compression plating of a fracture reduces and ______________ the fragments.

immobilizes

12 The rationale for using a compression plate is that the closer proximity of the fragments will speed up the union process because of stimulation of osteogenesis and because of the shorter distance that must be spanned by the callus. Clinical advantages are derived from the fact that neither traction nor a cast is needed to immobilize the fracture postoperatively; therefore, the patient is permitted to ambulate earlier. Compression plating speeds up the union process because ______________ is stimulated and the distance between the fragments is ______________.

osteogenesis
shorter

13 Compression plating is a variation of:

a. Traction
b. Metallic fixation
c. Reduction

b

14 Metallic fixation may be used to treat nonunion, delayed union, or malunion of fractures. After metallic fixation, the fracture may be further immobilized by the application of a cast or traction. List three approaches to immobilizing a fracture.

a. ______________________
b. ______________________
c. ______________________

a. Metallic fixation
b. Traction
c. Cast

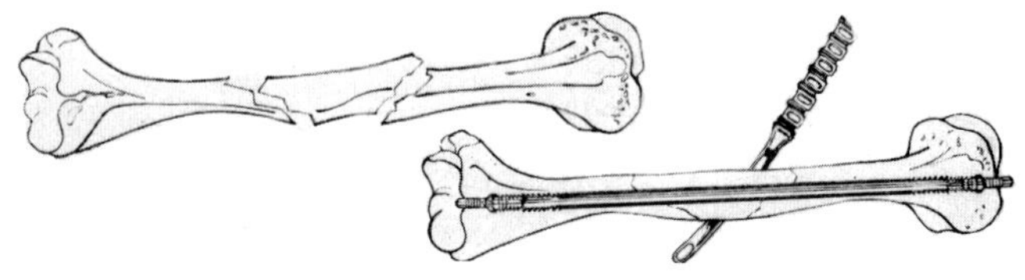

Fig. 6-4. An intramedullary rod has been inserted into the bone and a circumferential partial contact band is being placed around the bone to further immobilize the fragments. (Courtesy Richards Mfg. Co., Memphis.)

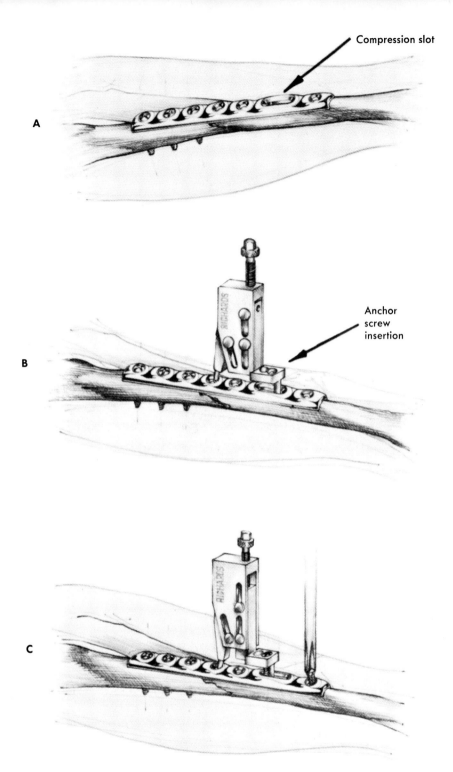

Fig. 6-5. A, Hirschhorn plate is secured to one side of the bone with screws. Note the compression slot between the two screw holes to the right of the fracture line. **B,** The compression device is in place over the plate with its foot in an appropriate screw hole. An anchor screw is placed through the plate compression slot on the opposite side of the fracture. **C,** The compression device is tightened with a special wrench until the fracture has been satisfactorily compressed. By pulling against the screw secured at left side of the fracture, the right side fragment slides to the left with the anchor screw moving along within the compression slot. Additional screws are then inserted and the anchor screw and compression device are removed. (Courtesy Richards Mfg. Co. Memphis.)

15 The fracture patient requiring open reduction and metallic fixation is often taken directly to surgery from the emergency department. Thus, the orthopedic nurse's first contact with the patient occurs after surgery. At the time of contact, the nurse assesses the patient's general status, the status of the operative site, and the status of the affected limb. Assessment of the patient's operative site may be somewhat impeded by the presence of a cast or traction. The surgical dressing restricts direct visualization of the wound; however, it can be examined for drainage and to ensure that it is intact. Immediate postoperative assessment of the patient after open reduction with metallic fixation includes:

a, b, c, d, and e

a. Listening to breath sounds
b. Taking vital signs
c. Measuring urinary output
d. Counting respiratory rate
e. Assessing pulse character
f. Measuring patient's height and weight

16 The circulatory and neuromuscular status and the position and alignment of the affected limb are determined as soon as possible after the patient is returned from surgery and periodically thereafter until the possibility of complications has decreased. The main circulatory functions to be assessed are extremity tissue perfusion and venous return. Tissue perfusion can be monitored by checking the extremity and by checking for nail bed blanching. (Nail bed blanching will be discussed in more detail in following chapters.) Immediate postoperative assessment focuses on the affected extremity's

circulatory; neuromuscular

position; alignment

_____ and _____ status and its _____ and _____ .

17 Checking of extremity pulse(s) distal to the fracture site provides

tissue perfusion

information regarding _____ .

skin color and temperature;
nail bed blanching

18 Other indications of tissue perfusion are _____
_____ and _____
_____ .

19 Assessment of circulatory status of the affected limb is directed

tissue perfusion

venous return

toward _____ and
_____ .

20 Neuromuscular function of the affected limb must be established

nerves; muscles

ligaments; tendons

because at the time of fracture _____ , _____ ,
_____ , or _____ may be injured.

58

asking him if can feel the
nurse's touch

21 Sensory function as reflected by patient's ability to perceive stimuli and pain demonstrates whether the nerves are intact. The nurse can test the patient's ability to perceive stimuli (in the affected limb) by _____

_____ .

22 Motor function is reflected by the patient's ability to move digits or to flex and extend the affected foot or arm (such movement may be restricted by a cast or traction). Assessment of the status of the affected extremity encompasses checking:

a. Tissue perfusion
b. Venous return
c. Sensory function
d. Motor function

a. _____

b. _____

c. _____

d. _____

23 The initial postoperative assessment can be subdivided into three major areas: _____ ,

general status

status of operative site

status of affected limb

_____ ,

and _____ .

24 Since the primary goal of orthopedic treatment is to restore normal function to the injured part, the nursing care plan should also focus on this goal. The incidents that cause fractures are traumatic emotionally as well as physically, and they create unique problems for each patient. Therefore, the patient's nursing care plan is comprised of the individual's unique problems and goals within a framework of the primary goal of treatment and the nursing actions for attaining those goals. The major objective of orthopedic nursing care is (to return the bone to normal size? to prevent infection? to assist the patient in resuming normal functioning?).

to assist the patient in
resuming normal functioning

25 The postoperative nursing care plan should emphasize the prevention of complications and continuous patient monitoring for indications of complications and response to treatment. Possible postoperative complications include, but are not limited to, hemorrhagic shock, atelectasis or pneumonia, thrombophlebitis, pulmonary embolus, fat embolus, urine retention, paralytic ileus, musculoskeletal problems, neurovascular damage, and infection. This list may seem overwhelmingly long but all of these are potential problems for most surgical patients. Therapeutic nursing interventions learned in relation to general surgical care can be directed toward prevention of most of these complications. The orthopedic nurse will tend to be more interested in the prevention or early recognition of musculoskeletal problems such as joint stiffness and contractures, joint subluxation or dislocation, foot drop, muscle atrophy, and possible breakage or dislodgement of the metallic fixation device. The major nursing care goals for the patient with open reduction and metallic fixation are:

a. To assist the patient to resume normal functioning
b. To prevent complications
c. To recognize complications early

a. _____

b. _____

c. _____

stiffness

contracture; subluxation

dislocation

26 The orthopedic nurse will be alert for musculoskeletal complications such as joint _____ , _____ , _____ , or _____ .

27 An activity plan and/or exercise routine should be initiated as soon as possible to assure that the nursing care goal of resuming normal functioning is attained. After metallic fixation, the patient should be encouraged to function as independently as possible. Simple movements of the joints above and below the fracture may be made if these joints are not included in the cast or traction. Such movements are essential to strengthen the muscles and to prevent joint stiffness or contractures that would limit functioning. Activity and exercises after metallic fixation prevent _____ _____ , _____ , and _____ .

muscle atrophy

joint stiffness

contractures

28 The most difficult aspect of caring for the metallic fixation patient, as well as other orthopedic patients, is deciding how to turn, move, and/or position the patient. It will be beneficial to think through what tissues have been surgically severed and sutured and relate this to changes that might accompany wound dehiscence. For example, when a femoral head prosthesis has been implanted to replace a severely fractured femoral head, the muscles holding the femoral head in the acetabulum have been cut and sutured. Thus a sudden sharp flexion of the hip joint might lead to breakage of the sutures and resultant subluxation or dislocation of the prosthesis. When turning, moving, or positioning an orthopedic patient, a general rule the nurse can follow is to _____ _____ _____ .

think through the surgical procedure and relate it to changes that might accompany wound dehiscence

29 Another general rule to be followed is to always maintain the prescribed degree of abduction or adduction or external or internal rotation of the involved extremity. If no specific instructions have been given, the nurse should check with the physician. Mr. Jones is to keep his legs abducted and the nurse is going to turn him on his side. While being turned, his legs must be kept in _____ .

abduction

30 The principles of body mechanics are applied in caring for the metallic fixation patient. One principle identified earlier was that the patient's joints are supported while an extremity is being moved. Mr. Smith has had an intramedullary pin inserted in his right femur and the nurse is moving him toward the edge of the bed in preparation for turning him. The nurse supports his right leg by _____

placing her hands under his right knee and ankle

31 It is more comfortable for the patient if the involved extremity is moved slowly and smoothly rather than with a quick, jerky motion. When turning Mr. Smith the nurse takes care to move his right leg _____ and _____ .

slowly; smoothly

32 Whenever any orthopedic patient is being turned, moved, lifted, or repositioned, it is essential that there be sufficient personnel available to ensure that adequate support of the affected extremity can be maintained and that the patient can be moved safely. The patient, when possible, should actively participate in the process. When turning Mr. Smith, the nurse protects his safety by _____

and by _____ .

getting other nursing personnel to help; having the patient help

33 The general rules to follow when moving, lifting, turning, or repositioning the patient after open reduction with metallic fixation are:

a. _____
b. _____
c. _____
d. _____
e. _____
f. _____

a. Think through surgical procedure.
b. Always maintain prescribed abduction/adduction or internal/external rotation.
c. Support joints of affected extremity.
d. Use slow, smooth movements.
e. Have enough assistance.
f. Involve patient in the process.

34 If a lower extremity fracture is not immobilized by traction, the patient may be permitted to walk with the use of crutches. Although the physical therapist may instruct the patient in the use of crutches, the nurse must encourage the patient and supervise him closely. Close supervision is required to prevent the patient from bearing weight on the affected extremity. The devices used in metallic fixation are _____ , _____ , _____ , and _____ .

pins; screws; nails; plates

35 Although intramedullary pins are quite strong, they can be broken when submitted to the stress of weight bearing before union occurs. The nurse supervises the crutch-walking patient after metallic fixation of the lower extremity primarily to prevent (accidents and poor posture? patient from bearing weight on the affected extremity? injury to his other leg?).

patient from bearing weight on the affected extremity

61

36 The use of medications in the treatment of fractures is usually limited to analgesics and antibiotics. Nursing care measures are used by the nurse as a means of relieving pain and enhancing the action of the analgesic. Some of the nursing care measures that can be used to relieve the orthopedic patient's discomfort include all of the following except:

c and e

a. Turning the patient
b. Talking with the patient
c. Asking all visitors to leave
d. Elevating the affected extremity (if appropriate)
e. Encouraging the patient to be quiet
f. Using diversionary materials to distract the patient
g. Encouraging activity or exercise

37 Mr. Jones is a 34-year-old man whose right femur was fractured in an auto accident 4 months ago. An intramedullary pin was inserted 2 days ago as treatment for nonunion. The patient has complained of pain. The nurse enters his room and sees that he is in semi-Fowler's position. What could the nurse do?

a. Talk with him
b. Change his position
c. Elevate his right leg
d. Give him an analgesic

a. _____
b. _____
c. _____
d. _____

38 As the nurse turns Mr. Jones, she talks with him and finds that he is accustomed to working with his hands and wants "something to do." How can this need be met?

a. By utilizing the resources available *(If available, occupational therapy could be requested.)*
b. By giving the patient a useful task to perform
c. By asking a family member to bring diversionary materials from home

a. _____
_____
b. _____
_____
c. _____
_____

39 The next day, the nurse watches as Mr. Jones walks down the hall on crutches. The nurse should watch him for all of the following except

a

a. To see that he doesn't leave the unit
b. To check his posture
c. To see if he is bearing weight on the right foot

40 In talking with patients, the nurse should always name the limb to which she is referring. Terms such as "good leg" and "bad leg" have connotations difficult to overcome. When Mr. Jones was first admitted 4 months ago, he was placed in traction (to prevent a fracture? infection? to reduce the fracture? to immobilize the fracture?).

to reduce the fracture, to immobilize the fracture

62

To assist him to resume normal functioning.

41 What is Mr. Jones' major nursing care goal?

42 Mrs. Brown fell and fractured the neck of her right femur. The orthopedist operated and used a Jewett nail and plate, as shown in Fig. 6-6, *A*, to immobilize the fragments. During the immediate postoperative phase of her hospitalization, Mrs. Brown's major nursing care goals are to _____ _____ and _____ _____ .

prevent complications; recognize as soon as possible complications that do occur

43 Which of the following general principles are applicable when turning Mrs. Brown?

a, c, and d

a. Move her smoothly and slowly.
b. Maintain abduction.
c. Involve patient in the process.
d. Relate knowledge of surgical procedure to possible complications.

44 The major rule for the nurse to remember when moving Mrs. Brown's right leg is to _____ _____ .

support the knee and ankle joints

45 Metallic fixation is the use of metallic devices to (reduce? immobilize?) a fracture.

immobilize

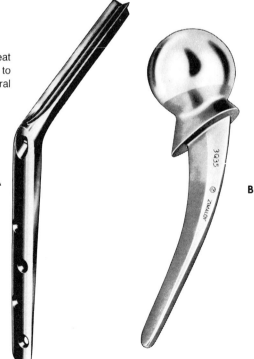

Fig. 6-6. A, Jewitt nail and plate combination used to treat fractured femoral neck; **B,** Thompson type prosthesis used to replace shattered femoral head and/or fractured femoral neck. (Courtesy Zimmer • USA, Warsaw, Ind.)

A

B

46 Metallic fixation immobilizes the (affected joint? surrounding muscles? bone fragments?).

47 Simple movements of the joints above and below the fracture are
a. Permitted if the joints are not in a cast
b. Not allowed
c. Permitted if the joints are not in traction

48 Metallic fixation and traction are used in the treatment of fractures (to increase the rate of union? to retain the desired position of the fragments until union occurs?).

49 The desired position of the fragments is attained by _____ .

50 The methods of reduction are (traction? closed reduction? metallic fixation? open reduction?).

51 After reduction, fractures are immobilized by all of the following except
a. Plaster casts
b. Sandbags
c. Traction
d. Metallic fixation
e. Intramedullary pin

52 Four types of metallic fixation devices are _____ , _____ , _____ , and _____ .

53 What is an intramedullary pin or nail?

54 After metallic fixation, nursing care measures can prevent musculoskeletal complications such as
a. _____
b. _____
c. _____
d. _____
e. _____
f. _____

55 The major foci of the initial postoperative assessment are:
_____ ,
_____ , and
_____ .

56 The status of the affected limb is determined by checking

circulatory and neuromuscular
functioning; position and
alignment of the affected
limb

_____

_____ and _____

_____ .

57 List three nursing care measures that could be taken to help relieve a patient's discomfort.

a. Change the patient's
position
b. Give the patient diversionary activity
c. Talk with patient
d. Elevate the affected
extremity
e. Encourage activity or
exercise
(Any three, any order)

a. _____

_____

b. _____

_____

c. _____

_____

Traction is the process of
pulling, either manually or
by a system of ropes,
pulleys, and weights.

58 What is traction?

59 Which of the following secondary goals could contribute to attainment of the major nursing care goal of the fracture patient?

All of these

a. To increase independence
b. To improve muscle strength of other extremities
c. To prevent contractures
d. To assist patient in finding vocational rehabilitation assistance

CHAPTER **7**

Principles of nursing care of the patient in traction

pulling force

1 *Traction* is the application of a pulling force to an area of the body or an extremity. The force may be obtained by pulling with the hands or by the pull of weights against a device connected to the patient. Weights or the hands may be used in order to exert a _____ _____ .

why the patient is in traction

2 Individualized care can be given to the patient in traction only when the nurse knows why the patient is in traction. The physician may prescribe traction in the treatment of fractures, injuries to the musculoskeletal system, and inflammatory conditions. Although the specific rationale underlying the physician's selection of traction as the method of treatment may not be known, it can be inferred from the patient's diagnosis. Before caring for the patient in traction, the nurse must know _____ _____ .

reduced; immobilized

3 Traction is most frequently prescribed in the treatment of fractures. Traction may be utilized to reduce and/or immobilize the fracture. By exerting a pulling force on the affected part in some types of fractures, the bone fragments can be realigned. Traction is employed in the treatment of fractures so that the fracture may be _____ and/or _____ .

muscles

4 Immobilization of the fracture maintains the position of the bone fragments. In Chapter 6 it was noted that the position of the reduced fracture must be maintained to assure that the fragments heal in the aligned position. In addition, fragment motion must be restricted since it could stimulate muscle spasms. Fractures are immobilized by traction in order to control the position of the bone fragments and thereby prevent stimulation of the _____ .

traction

5 Traction immobilization may be indicated both before and after a fracture has been reduced. Before reduction, traction immobilization may relieve or prevent muscle spasms. The muscle spasms associated with a fracture can be extremely painful; however, they can be relieved or prevented by the application of _____ .

66

6 After reduction, even the slightest fragment motion may be sufficient to stimulate muscle spasms, and the muscle spasms could pull the fracture out of alignment. Muscle spasms caused by fragment motion must be prevented after reduction because _____ _____ and _____ _____.

they are painful; they can pull the fracture out of alignment

7 When traction is utilized to immobilize and/or reduce a fracture, movement of the joint above and the joint below the fracture must be prevented. Joint immobilization of the fractured limb ensures prevention of _____ motion.

fragment

8 Fragment motion in a reduced fracture is undesirable because _____ _____ and because _____ _____.

muscle spasms can be stimulated; fragments can be pulled out of alignment

9 Traction may be prescribed as the method of treating other injuries to the musculoskeletal system for the same reasons that it is used in the treatment of fractures; muscle spasms can be _____ and/or _____.

prevented; relieved

10 Traction may be indicated to correct and maintain skeletal alignment, not only for treatment of fractures but also when a bone has been dislocated. Emergency treatment of a dislocated shoulder, for example, includes application of traction by attaching a bucket of water to the involved extremity while the sedated patient lies prone, as shown in Fig. 7-1. Traction is used to reduce _____ and _____.

fractures

dislocations

11 In some instances traction may be employed to inhibit or reduce post-trauma edema such as might be encountered with a badly sprained ankle. Although immobilization with other means is more commonly utilized, traction may be employed to obtain the benefits of immobilization and elevation of the involved extremity since it will _____.

inhibit or reduce edema

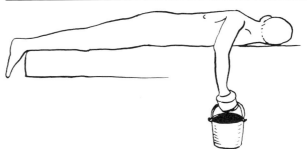

Fig. 7-1. Application of a pulling force to treat a shoulder dislocation.

12 When a wound is infected, traction may be applied to elevate the limb to facilitate wound drainage. As in the treatment of traumatic injuries, traction may be used in the treatment of wound infections because the traction apparatus _____ the limbs.

elevates

13 Traction relieves muscle spasms by exerting a pulling force greater than the pull of the contracting muscles. Therefore, it is also used as a means of preventing and/or correcting deformities associated with muscle contraction. The physician may prescribe traction in order to _____ and/or _____ a fracture or to _____ and/or _____ a deformity.

reduce; immobilize
prevent; correct

14 Traction immobilization is used in the treatment of inflammatory conditions in order to permit a joint to heal or rest. In these conditions, the amount of traction (pulling force) may be minimal since muscle spasms are not the primary indication for traction. Before caring for a patient in traction, the nurse should identify the rationale underlying the use of traction for that specific patient. Mr. Jones has an inflammatory condition in his right hip and has been placed in traction since the physician does not want him to bear weight on the joint. The nurse may infer from this brief description that traction is being utilized _____ _____ .

to permit the inflamed hip
joint to rest

15 One universal purpose of traction is to help correct and maintain skeletal alignment. This includes the use of traction to reduce and/or immobilize fractures and dislocations and to prevent or correct deformities. Any time that traction is utilized, the physician applies the pulling force in a specific therapeutic direction; that is, the traction force pulls in a direction that will bring about the desired skeletal alignment. The primary goal of traction is:

c
a. To exert force
b. To reduce a fracture
c. To exert a pulling force
d. To prevent deformity

16 Match the two sets of terms to complete the reasons for using traction.

c, d   ____ 1. Reduce   a. Joint
a   ____ 2. Permit healing   b. Deformity
b   ____ 3. Prevent   c. Fracture
a   ____ 4. Permit rest   d. Dislocations
b   ____ 5. Correct
c   ____ 6. Immobilize

17 The four basic traction types are manual, skin, skeletal, and encircling. In skin, manual, and encircling traction, the pulling force is transmitted to the affected part indirectly through the skin. The basic traction types are _____, _____, _____, and _____.

manual; skin
skeletal; encircling

18 As the name implies, in manual traction the hands are used to exert a pulling force. Manual traction may be instituted by the nurse as an emergency or temporary measure until one of the other methods can be applied. Manual traction can be used:

a, c, and d

a. While skin traction equipment is being prepared
b. When assisting in the removal of a plaster cast
c. As a first aid measure after an accident
d. When a traction rope breaks

19 Skin traction exerts a pulling force on the extremity through adherent straps and bandages applied to the skin. The adherent straps may be foam-rubber backed cloth straps that tend to cling to the skin or strips of adhesive tape. A simple system of ropes, pulleys,

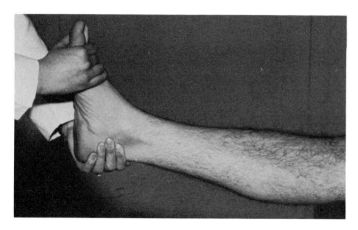

Fig. 7-2. The application of manual traction.

Fig. 7-3. Skin traction applied to the lower leg. (Courtesy Zimmer · USA, Warsaw, Ind.)

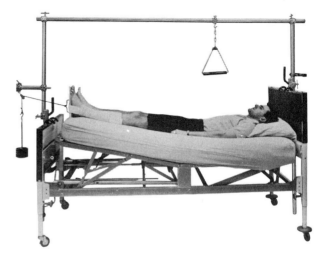

69

and weights is connected to the adherent straps to attain a pulling force. Manual and skin traction are similar because the pulling force is transmitted to the affected part through the _____ .

skin

20 Skin traction is often used as a temporary means of immobilizing a fracture until an open reduction can be performed. Skin traction is applied by (grasping firmly with the hands? bandages and slings? attaching adherent straps to the skin?).

attaching adherent
straps to the skin

21 Skin traction is impractical over long periods of time because the skin beneath the adherent straps tends to become excoriated and because the bandages may cause pressure sores. Skin traction is used as a (first aid? long-term? short-term?) measure.

short-term

22 Skin traction cannot be continued for weeks or months because:

c

a. The patient must be allowed up.
b. The patient will heal without it.
c. The patient's skin will break down.
d. The adherent straps will come loose.

23 Skeletal traction is applied by inserting a metal device such as a Kirschner wire, Steinmann pin, or Kranendonk pin through the bone. The Kirschner wire is threaded like a screw, while the Steinmann pin is unthreaded. The Kranendonk modified skeletal traction pin is a unique combination of the Kirschner wire and the Steinmann pin in that it is unthreaded except for a small portion, which is used to firmly secure the pin into the cortex of the bone. All of these are made of stainless steel — allergic reactions are rare. In skeletal traction, the wire or pin is connected to the system of ropes and pulleys and the traction or pulling force is applied to the _____ .

bone

24 One advantage of skin traction is that the skin surface is not broken, thus reducing the possibility of infection. The disadvantages of skeletal traction by pin insertion include _____ .

infection

25 The patient is able to tolerate skeletal traction over an extended period of time because the pulling force is transmitted directly to the bone rather than to the skin. When anchored firmly in the bone, the skeletal traction pin or wire is not uncomfortable for the patient. However, if the pin or wire slips from side to side through the bone, as may occur if the pin tract becomes infected, the patient may experience pain. Skeletal traction can be used for (lengthy? short?) periods of time.

lengthy

26 Skeletal traction is tolerated over longer periods of time because the pulling force is applied directly to the bone, and this allows greater amounts of weight to be utilized. Also, the traction can be

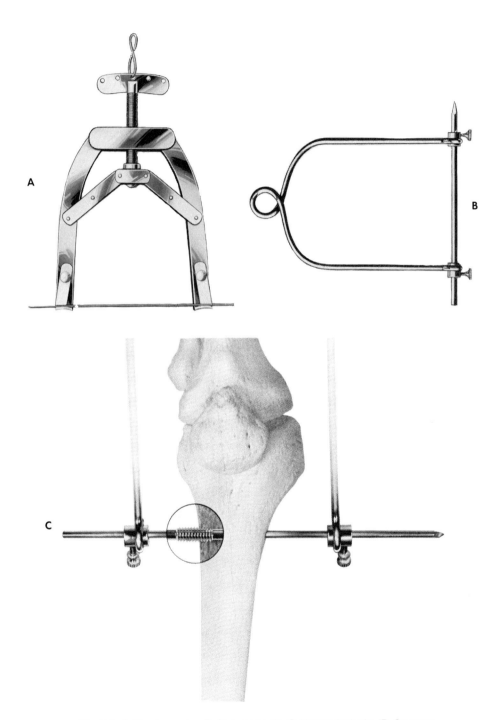

Fig. 7-4. A, Kirschner wire, **B,** Steinmann pin, **C,** Kranendonk pin. (**B,** Courtesy Zimmer • USA, Warsaw, Ind.; **C,** courtesy Richards Mfg. Co., Memphis.)

applied more accurately. The advantages of skeletal over skin traction include:

a, b, d, and e

a. More weight can be applied.

b. Skeletal traction can be tolerated longer.

c. Skin becomes excoriated in a short period of time.

d. Traction can be applied more accurately.

e. The patient is more comfortable.

27 Skeletal traction is used primarily in the treatment of fractures of long bones. Skeletal traction via Crutchfield, Barton, or Vinke tongs placed in the skull is used in the treatment of cervical spine fractures, and nursing care of these patients requires knowledge of neurology as well as orthopedics. Mr. Smith is admitted with a fractured right femur. The physician is likely to prescribe _____ traction.

skeletal

28 On the basis of your knowledge of bone healing rates, briefly describe why the physician is likely to prescribe skeletal traction for Mr. Smith.

The long bones require a longer period of time to heal than other bones and therefore must be immobilized longer. The patient can tolerate skeletal traction over an extended period of time.

29 The methods of applying traction are _____, _____, _____, and _____.

manual

skin; skeletal; encircling

30 Traction may also be applied by encircling an extremity or part of the body with a special device such as a pelvic traction belt. *Encircling* traction is considered by some to be a form of skin traction because the encircling device transmits the pulling force to the skin. The traction methods that transmits their pulling force through the skin are _____, _____, and _____.

manual; skin; encircling

Fig. 7-5. Skeletal traction applied by inserting a Kirschner wire into the distal end of the femur. (Courtesy Zimmer · USA, Warsaw, Ind.)

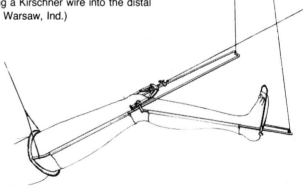

31 To obtain the prescribed amount of traction, the device that has been attached to the patient is connected to a system of ropes, pulleys, and weights using a metal frame on the bed. The physician's prescription should specify the amount of traction (weight in pounds) and whether the traction is to be *continuous* or *intermittent*. Some forms of skin and encircling tractions may be used on an intermittent basis; the traction may be removed periodically. When the traction can be removed at intervals, it is referred to as _____ traction.

intermittent

32 *Continuous* traction must remain in place at all times until the physician removes it. Continuous traction is typically applied in the treatment of fractures. If the traction is not to be removed, the physician's order will indicate that the traction is to be _____.

continuous

33 Well-meaning persons may mistakenly remove continuous traction in the belief that it is the source of the patient's discomfort. However, premature removal of continuous traction from a fractured extremity can have serious consequences for the patient since bone fragment motion may occur. Bone fragment motion is undesirable because a progressively damaging and painful cycle may be generated. The fragments may stimulate the muscles resulting in muscle spasms that are painful and may serve to pull the bone fragments out of alignment and lead to even more severe muscle spasms. The fragments may also sever blood vessels or nerves. Mr. Black is in continuous skeletal traction for treatment of his fractured femur. He complains of pain and asks the nurse to remove the traction. The nurse (should? should not?) remove the traction.

should not

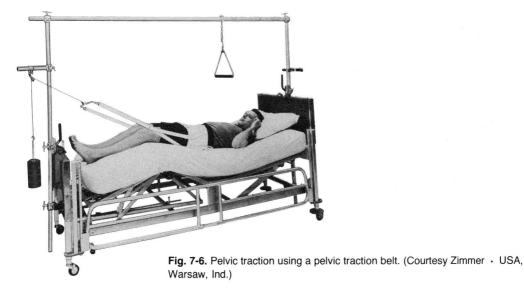

Fig. 7-6. Pelvic traction using a pelvic traction belt. (Courtesy Zimmer · USA, Warsaw, Ind.)

34 In many hospitals all of the traction equipment is kept in one room or on a cart, and an attendant or orthopedic technician is responsible for the equipment and assists the physician. Traction is used in the treatment of orthopedic conditions to (immobilize a fracture? relieve pain? increase the rate of union? relax muscles?).

immobilize a fracture,
relieve pain, relax muscles

35 The physician should perform the initial application of the pulling force because it can result in a severe and potentially damaging episode of muscle spasms. The muscle spasms could be particularly damaging if traction is being used to treat a fracture because the fracture fragments could sever a blood vessel or nerve. The nurse assembles the equipment, prepares the patient, and assists the physician in the application of traction. What traction method may be used in the process of applying skin traction? _____

manual traction

36 The skin must be clean and dry before skin traction is applied. If painful removal of the adherent straps is anticipated, the hair on the extremity may be trimmed prior to the application of traction. The nurse prepares the patient's skin by (wiping it with alcohol? washing it? drying it? powdering it? shaving it?).

washing it, drying it
*(Shaving is incorrect; doing
so may irritate the skin.)*

37 In skin traction the adherent straps are applied to both sides of the extremity, and an elastic bandage is wrapped over them to hold them in place. The ends of the adherent straps are then attached to a spreader to which the remainder of the traction system has been connected. The equipment needed to apply skin traction includes:

a, b, c, e, f, and g

a. Ropes   e. Weights
b. Pulleys   f. Elastic bandages
c. Spreader   g. Adherent straps
d. Steinmann pin

38 The bandages over the adherent straps must be loose enough to prevent impairment of circulation and tight enough to afford good contact. The bandages should be rewrapped periodically to prevent pressure areas from developing. If the skin traction is to be applied to the lower extremity, the spreader must be as wide as the patient's ankle to prevent the straps from putting pressure on the malleoli. List four possible complications related to the use of skin traction.

a. Development of pressure
   areas from the bandages
b. Skin excoriation under the
   bandages
c. Pressure areas on the
   malleoli
d. Circulatory impairment

a. _____

b. _____

c. _____

d. _____

39 The physician determines the amount and location of the weights attached to the system of ropes and pulleys. For leg traction the size

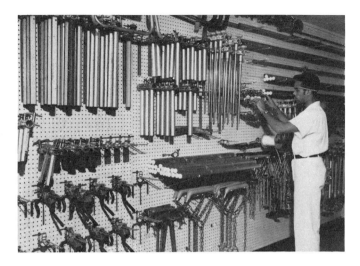

Fig. 7-7. The orthopedic technician in the traction equipment room at The Ohio State University Hospitals, Columbus, Ohio.

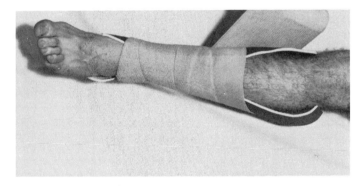

Fig. 7-8. The application of adhesive straps to both sides of the extremity.

Fig. 7-9. The spreader is wider than the ankle.

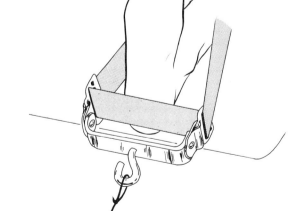

of the spreader is determined by the _____

size of the patient's ankle _____ . The spreader must be wider

prevent pressure areas than the ankle to _____ .

40 Some forms of skin traction are called *running* or *straight traction,* since in the simpler forms, such as Buck's extension, the trac-

skin tion force is in a straight line. Buck's extension is a form of (skin? skeletal?) traction.

41 Skin traction is like encircling traction because the traction force that is transmitted to the muscles and bones is applied to the

skin _____ .

42 Pelvic and cervical traction are two common forms of encircling traction. In each, a device is placed around a part of the body and weight is attached with the force in a straight line. The traction force

Buck's extension is also in a straight line in _____
traction.

43 To apply cervical and pelvic traction, a spreader bar, rope, pulleys, and weights and either a pelvic traction belt or head halter will be needed. If bilateral Buck's extension were applied to the

would patient's legs, it (would? would not?) serve the same purpose as pelvic traction.

44 Bilateral Buck's extension traction is like pelvic traction because

pull in a straight line; trans- they both _____

mit their pulling forces
to the skin _____ and _____

_____ .

Fig. 7-10. A, Pelvic traction belt; **B,** cervical traction head halter. (Courtesy
Zimmer · USA, Warsaw, Ind.)

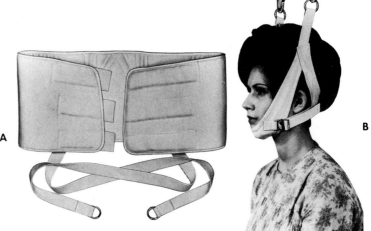

A

B

45 Pelvic, 90-90 pelvic, or Buck's extension traction may be prescribed to treat low back pain. When traction is applied in the treatment of low back pain, the purpose of the traction is to flatten the lumbar curve by pulling on the lower back. This approach tends to relieve pressure on the sciatic nerve, which is often involved in low back pain. The types of traction employed in the treatment of

pelvic; 90-90

Buck's extension

low back pain are _____, _____, and _____ .

46 Traction used for the treatment of low back pain may be applied and/or removed by the nurse or patient according to the physician's instructions. Often, the physician will order the patient to be in traction "as tolerated." Traction applied for 1 hour four times a day is

intermittent

referred to as _____ traction.

47 Russell's traction is similar to Buck's extension except that a sling is added to support the knee. Use of a knee sling also alters the direction of the traction force (Fig. 7-12). The physician moves the knee sling pulley caudad or cephalad to obtain the desired traction force direction. For Russell's traction, Buck's traction is modified

knee sling

by the addition of a _____ .

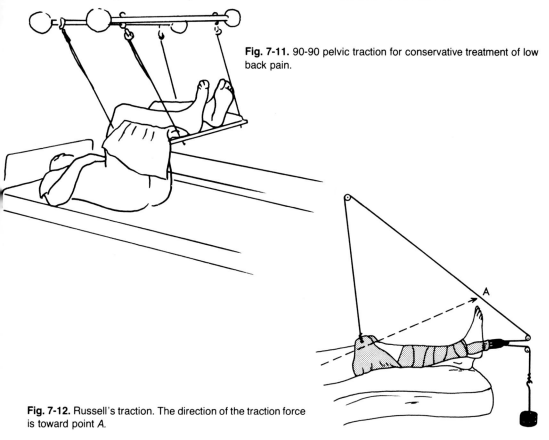

Fig. 7-11. 90-90 pelvic traction for conservative treatment of low back pain.

Fig. 7-12. Russell's traction. The direction of the traction force is toward point *A*.

changes the direction of the traction pull, supports the knee

48 In Russell's traction, the sling under the patient's knee (holds the knee in place? changes the direction of the traction pull? supports the knee?).

49 Complete the following:

Devices used to apply traction	Name of method
Adherent straps	_____
Hands	_____
Pelvic traction belt	_____
Kirschner wire	_____

Skin
Manual
Encircling
Skeletal

50 The physician inserts the Kirschner wire or Steinmann pin using sterile technique to prevent a bone infection. A U shaped spreader is clamped onto the pin or wire and attached to the system of ropes, pulleys, and weights. Pins and wires are inserted using sterile technique in order to _____ .

prevent bone infection

51 Before the wire on pin is inserted, it is much longer than necessary for attaching the spreader. The physician will cut off one end of the wire or pin after it is in place. The pin is shortened so that it will not come into contact with the splint or Pearson attachment. The spreaders used for skeletal traction and for skin traction are (alike? different?).

different

52 Care must be exercised to avoid accidental contact with the protruding pin ends, since this would be uncomfortable for the pa-

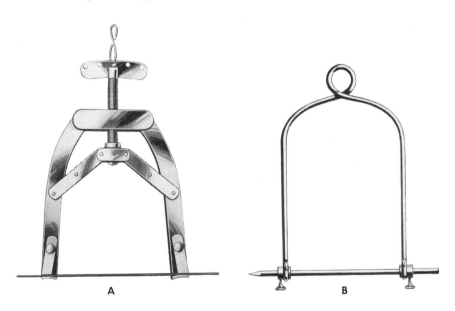

Fig. 7-13. A, Kirschner wire tractor; **B,** Böhler-Steinmann pin holder. (Courtesy Zimmer · USA, Warsaw, Ind.)

tient. Also, the pin ends tend to be sharp and could cause injury; therefore, corks or protective plastic caps should be placed over the pin ends. Since contact with the protruding pin ends may cause fragment motion, the patient's resultant discomfort may be due to

muscle spasms
_____ .

53 Skeletal traction is frequently combined with a complex system of ropes, pulleys, and supportive devices. The *balanced suspension* system is designed to support the affected extremity, maintain the desired direction of the pulling force, and maintain the desired degree of abduction. Balanced suspension of the affected limb permits freedom of movement of the remainder of the body and facilitates nursing care, since the patient can be lifted off the bed without disturbing the angle or direction of the pulling force. The purposes underlying the use of balanced suspension are to:

a. Support the affected extremity
b. Maintain desired direction of the pulling force
c. Maintain desired degree of abduction

a. _____
_____

b. _____
_____

c. _____
_____

The advantages associated with the use of balanced suspension traction are:

d. Permits freedom of movement
e. Facilitates nursing care

d. _____

e. _____

54 A balanced suspension system may be used without skeletal traction to elevate or support an extremity after surgery. In suspen-

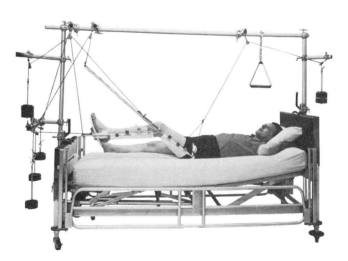

Fig. 7-14. Balanced skeletal traction, the leg is suspended in a Thomas leg splint with a Pearson attachment. (Courtesy Zimmer • USA, Warsaw, Ind.)

79

sion, a Thomas splint or similar hammock-like device is used to support the limb in the desired position. The splint is then suspended by a system of ropes, pulleys, and weights. A Thomas splint is used

elevate; support

to _____ and/or _____ the affected leg.

55 A Pearson attachment is often used with a Thomas splint or Keller-Blake splint so that the leg may be positioned with the knee flexed. Suspension traction maintains the affected limb in a(n)

specific, therapeutic

(adducted? specific? therapeutic?) position.

56 If a Thomas splint, a Pearson attachment, and a Kirschner wire are used, there are two sets of ropes, pulleys, and weights. One set

skeletal traction

is for the _____ system and

balanced suspension

the other is for the _____ system.

pulling

57 The skeletal traction system applies the _____

desired direction of the pulling force; desired degree of abduction

force. The balanced suspension system maintains the _____

_____

_____ and the _____

_____ .

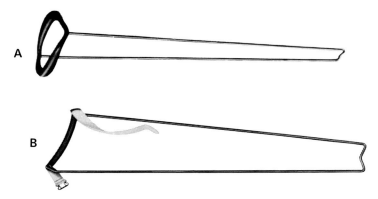

Fig. 7-15. A, Full ring Thomas leg splint; **B,** half ring Thomas leg splint. (Courtesy Zimmer · USA, Warsaw, Ind.)

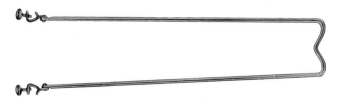

Fig. 7-16. Pearson attachment for Thomas leg splint. (Courtesy Zimmer · USA, Warsaw, Ind.)

58 The patient has had surgery on his right hip and the physician has requested a Thomas splint and a Pearson attachment. It appears that the physician is going to use the balanced suspension to:
a. Pull the affected limb into a prescribed position
b. Support the affected limb in a therapeutic position
c. Maintain the affected limb in a therapeutic position
d. Maintain the prescribed direction of the pulling force

59 Skeletal traction and balanced suspension are used together in the treatment of a fractured extremity (never? sometimes? always?).

60 For traction to be effective, an equal amount of pull must be exerted against the traction weights. *Countertraction* is essential to keep the patient from being pulled against the pulleys, negating the traction force. Countertraction is a pulling force _____ and _____ the traction weights.

61 Countertraction can be obtained by tilting the bed in the opposite direction of the traction. Without countertraction, the traction force (will? will not?) be effective.

62 Countertraction is necessary:
a. To prevent the patient from being pulled toward the pulleys
b. To keep the equipment in line
c. For the traction to accomplish its purpose
d. To prevent negation of the traction force

63 Miss Gray, an 80-year-old, 100-pound retired schoolteacher, fell on the ice this morning and has been admitted with a fractured left femoral neck. The physician has placed 10 pounds of Buck's extension traction on her left leg. Soon afterward, the nurse finds Miss Gray pulled down toward the foot of the bed. The nurse:
a. Reports her observation to her supervisor
b. Checks to see if the spreader bar is against the pulley
c. Recognizes that Miss Gray is too thin for traction to be effective
d. Asks her team leader for assistance in pulling Miss Gray up in bed

64 The nurse found that the spreader bar was resting on the pulley and recognized that if Miss Gray was pulled up in bed she would slide down again unless some measure was taken to prevent it. The nurse realized that _____ was necessary.

65 To obtain countertraction, the nurse could:
a. Put a restraining jacket on Miss Gray
b. Apply 10 pounds of cervical traction
c. Elevate the foot of the bed on shock blocks

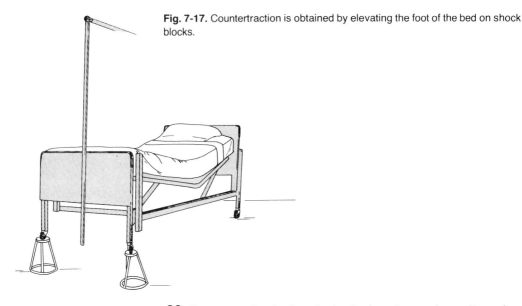

Fig. 7-17. Countertraction is obtained by elevating the foot of the bed on shock blocks.

equal to, against

66 Countertraction is also obtained when the traction pulls against a fixed point. When a Thomas splint is used, the ring presses against the ischial tuberosity, which is the fixed point. The Thomas splint provides a pulling force (greater than? equal to? against? in same direction as?) the traction weights.

pulley

67 The effect of the traction is reduced if the rope is in contact with the bed or covers, if the patient's extremity is pressing against the bed, and if the spreader is resting on the bed or _____ .

manual traction

68 If a traction rope breaks, the nurse could apply _____ _____ until the rope is replaced.

a, b, and d

69 The nursing care of a patient in traction includes frequent observations of the traction equipment, such as:
a. Checking for frayed and worn ropes
b. Checking the spreader's location and size
c. Checking whether the patient has remained in traction
d. Checking whether the bed covers have become tangled in the traction rope

c

70 The physician prescribes the amount of weight that is applied. On each tour of duty the nurse should verify that the prescribed amount is in place. The prescribed amount of weight is effective only when it is hanging free and is not in contact with the bed, floor, or equipment. As she makes rounds, the nurse finds that Mr. Jones has 25 pounds of weight instead of the prescribed 20 pounds. The nurse should:
a. Remove the extra 5 pounds and notify the physician immediately

b. Leave the weight in place and notify the physician when he comes in the next day

c. Leave the weight in place and notify the physician immediately

71 Mr. Smith's right leg is suspended in a Thomas ring splint. The nurse notices that the foot of his bed is not elevated on shock blocks. The nurse remembers that:

a. Countertraction is provided by the ring pressing on the ischial tuberosity.

b. Countertraction is not needed.

c. Countertraction is obtained by pulling against a fixed point.

72 Proper body alignment is essential for the traction patient to prevent deformity and to maintain the prescribed position of the extremity in traction. If the traction is arranged so that the patient's leg appears to be in abduction, abduction (should? should not?) be maintained.

73 The nurse is checking the traction equipment as shown in Fig. 7-18. What needs to be corrected?

(The changes from removal could be as damaging as they are when traction is applied.)

a and c

should
(Check with the physician when in doubt.)

The weights are resting on the bed.

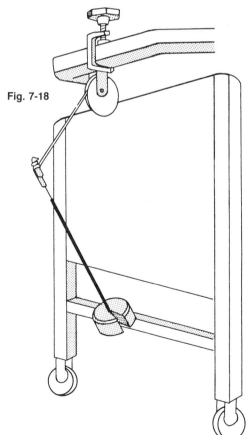

Fig. 7-18

74 The physician may arrange the traction apparatus with the affected extremity in abduction or adduction. This position must be maintained. Sandbags, foot boards, or other devices may be used to maintain the position. The physician has applied 20 pounds of skeletal traction to the patient's right leg, which is suspended in a Thomas splint and abducted. Indicate which positions are correct and which are incorrect.

_____ a. The patient has moved so his legs are adducted.

_____ b. The patient has his left leg flexed and his right leg abducted.

_____ c. The patient has both legs abducted.

75 The traction patient's body alignment is important because:

a. The proper alignment (position) maintains the direction of the pulling force.
b. The proper position can prevent the traction from pulling correctly.
c. The proper position prevents the development of deformities.

76 The nurse should look at the traction patient's extremities to ascertain whether the prescribed degree of abduction is being maintained. If the limb in traction is to be abducted, the nurse should look at its position in relation to _____

_____ .

77 Abduction or adduction of the traction patient's extremities can be maintained by the placement of _____ , _____

_____ , or _____ .

78 While caring for the patient in traction, the nurse should check the patient and the traction equipment for:

a. Friction on the traction ropes
b. Proper method of traction
c. Proper body alignment
d. Progress in healing of fracture
e. Correct amount of weight
f. Effective countertraction

79 The type of traction apparatus, the prescribed direction of the pulling force, the location of the affected extremity or body part, and the source of countertraction determine the body positions the patient can assume. The prescribed direction of the pulling force and the countertraction must be maintained. The factors that determine whether the patient can be placed in Fowler's position or turn to his side are:

a. _____

b. Prescribed direction of the
   pulling force
c. Location of the affected
   extremity or part
d. Source of countertraction

b. _____

c. _____

d. _____

80 Most types of traction on either or both of the lower extremities tend to preclude use of the prone and side-lying positions. Indicate which of the following factors should be considered when a patient with Buck's extension traction on his right leg requests to turn on his right side:

a and b

a. The pull of the traction is in a straight line.
b. Countertraction is provided by the patient's body weight.
c. Pressure on the injury or operative site should be avoided.
d. The position of the left leg must be maintained.

81 If the patient with traction on a lower extremity is permitted to sit in a Fowler's position, the effect of the traction may be lessened because of the loss of countertraction. When countertractoin is obtained from pulling against a fixed point, elevation of the head of the bed is permitted unless precluded by some other factor. The source of countertraction (is? is not?) a determinant of whether the head of the traction patient's bed may be elevated.

is

82 The patient with balanced suspension and skeletal traction on the lower extremity is restricted by the traction equipment and cannot lie on his side or abdomen. The patient's right leg is supported by a Thomas splint. If he attempts to turn to his right side:

a and c

a. The splint and ropes will be in the way.
b. The nurse should place a pillow behind his back.
c. The prescribed degree of abduction will be lost.

83 The patient with traction on an upper extremity is restricted in the positions that he may assume. When considering how the patient may be positioned, the nurse should remember that the _____

prescribed direction of the
pulling force; counter-
traction

_____ and _____ must be maintained.

84 The other two factors that determine how the patient can be positioned are:

a. Type of traction apparatus
b. Location of the affected
   extremity or body part

a. _____
   _____

b. _____
   _____

85 While caring for the patient in traction, the nurse should check that the *patient's position* in bed

a. Maintains the prescribed
   direction of the pulling force

a. _____

b. Maintains the prescribed abduction of the affected extremity

c. Maintains effective countertraction

d. Prevents development of deformities

b. _____

c. _____

d. _____

86 While caring for the patient in traction, the nurse should check the *traction equipment* to verify that:

a. Prescribed amount of weight is in use

b. Traction ropes are in good condition

c. Weights are hanging freely

d. Traction ropes are not in contact with the bed or linens

e. Spreader is not resting on a pulley

a. _____

b. _____

c. _____

d. _____

e. _____

87 The condition of the skin and the circulation to the extremity in traction must be checked frequently. Indications of circulatory impairment and skin reactions should be reported to the physician. Indications of circulatory disturbances include changes in the skin

color; temperature
_____ and _____ .

88 When Russell's traction or a Thomas splint and Pearson attachment are used, pressure on the head of the fibula from contact with the sling or attachment may lead to peroneal nerve damage. Contact with the splint or Pearson attachment on the lateral aspect of the

peroneal nerve damage
upper calf may cause _____ .

89 When a sling, support, or encircling device is used, it should be checked frequently and any wrinkles or ridges removed. At the same time, the portion of the patient's skin that is in contact with the sling or support must be checked for indications of irritation or the formation of pressure areas. The nurse should also check the

circulatory impairment
nerve damage
extremity in traction for indications of _____
_____ and _____ .

90 The nurse checks the extremity in traction for indications of

circulatory impairment; nerve damage; pressure areas
_____ , _____
_____ , and _____ .

91 When a Thomas splint, with or without a Pearson attachment, is used, the Achilles tendon, the groin, and the ischial tuberosity should be checked for signs of pressure and skin irritation. The ischial tuberosity is prone to the development of pressure areas since it provides the fixed point for countertraction. After checking the patient who has his right leg in a Thomas splint with a Pearson attachment, which of the following would the nurse report to the physician?

b, c, and d

a. The patient's right foot is warm and pink.
b. The patient has an excoriated area in his groin.
c. The toes of the right foot are cold and cyanotic.
d. The patient complains of a tingling sensation in his right foot.

92 The skin over the groin area and the ischial tuberosity should be moved from under the splint periodically to relieve the pressure. The nurse should observe all traction patients for indications of complications such as _____,

circulatory impairment; skin reactions; pressure areas; nerve damage

_____ , _____

_____ , and _____ .

93 Pressure areas and skin irritation can develop under or at the edge of the traction device or equipment. The skin in these areas must be checked frequently and skin care given as needed. Complete the following table:

Type of traction	Skin points to be checked
Russell's traction	a. _____
Skeletal traction	b. _____
(Thomas splint)	c. _____
	d. _____
	e. _____
Pelvic traction	f. _____

a. Posterior aspect of knee
b. Achilles tendon
c. Posterior aspect of leg
d. Groin
e. Ischial tuberosity
   (b through e, any order)
f. Iliac crests

94 The traction apparatus used on any part of the lower extremity should include a means of supporting the foot. Although the patient may be able to move the foot and exercise it, foot drop may still develop unless the foot is supported in the correct position. The correct anatomical name for foot drop position is _____

plantar flexion

_____ .

95 The nurse checking a traction patient's skin is checking for signs of _____ , _____

skin irritation; pressure areas (or sores); circulatory impairment

_____ , and _____ .

96 The nurse checks the slings and supports for _____

wrinkles

ridges
(any source of pressure)

and _____ .

97 Preventable complications for the traction patient include

_____ , _____ , _____ , _____ , and _____ .

98 The skin points that must be checked for indications of pressure area development when Buck's extension traction is being used include the instep and Achilles tendon of the foot in traction and the heels of both feet. The elastic bandages tend to develop wrinkles that can impair circulation or lead to the development of pressure areas. The skin checkpoints to be checked (do? do not?) vary with the type of traction being used.

do

99 The skin checkpoints for the patient in Buck's extension traction include (heels? knees? Achilles tendon? instep?).

heels, Achilles tendon, instep

100 The methods of applying traction are: _____ , _____ , _____ , and _____ .

manual

skin; skeletal; encircling

101 Skeletal traction is applied by _____ _____ .

inserting a metal device into the bone

102 The nursing care of the patient in skeletal traction should include periodic observations of the skin at both ends of the pin or wire. The area should be checked for signs of infection. Any drainage, foul odor, or swelling at the pin site should be reported to the physician. Additional observations about the extremity in traction that the nurse should report are:

a. Patient complaints of numbness or tingling

a, c, and d

b. Warm skin temperature

c. Discoloration of skin (for example, redness)

d. Swelling

103 The skin at both ends of a Kirschner wire should be checked periodically for signs of _____ .

infection

104 The indications of infection of the pin site are (edema? purulent drainage? numbness? foul odor?).

edema, purulent drainage, foul odor

105 The traction patient has many of the problems that other bedridden patients have. In addition to the pressure sores from contact with the traction apparatus, the patient may also develop decubiti over those areas that are constantly subjected to friction and pressure, such as the coccyx, elbows, and heels. As long as the traction pull is not disturbed, the patient may be lifted so that skin care can be given to the coccyx. The area should be massaged with powder, corn starch, or lotion, whichever is appropriate for the patient. Problems common to most traction patients are (elimination? prevention of decubiti? nutrition? relief of pain?).

106 Pressure on the elbows and heels can be relieved by the use of padding such as foam rubber, sheet wadding, and protective devices made for this purpose. Massaging with lotion is also helpful. When the patient is in Russell's traction, decubiti on the coccyx can be prevented by:

b, c, and d
a. Removing the traction and turning the patient
b. Providing a "sheepskin" pad for the patient to sit on
c. Lifting the patient up and rubbing the coccyx
d. Keeping the bed free of wrinkles

107 When the patient is in traction, the areas of his body that are

heels; coccyx; elbows; scapula or other bony prominences
prone to the formation of decubiti are _____ , _____ , _____ , and _____ _____ .

108 Which nursing care measures help to prevent decubiti on the elbows and heels?

a, b, and c
(In some hospitals, "donuts" are not permitted as they are thought to cut off circulation.)
a. Massaging the area
b. Rubbing the area with lotion
c. Wrapping the elbows with sheet wadding
d. Placing a "donut" under the heel

skin traction
109 Encircling traction is similar to _____ .

constant
110 Unless otherwise indicated, traction is (intermittent? constant?).

111 For the traction to be effective, there must be an opposite and equal force against it. The opposite and equal force is

countertraction
_____ .

112 Skin traction is applied by:

c
a. Pulling with the hands
b. Applying a pelvic traction belt
c. Attaching adhesive straps to the extremity

113 The physician calls and tells the nurse that Mr. Johnson is being admitted with a fractured right femur and that the nurse should have the equipment ready to apply Buck's extension traction. The equipment the nurse should assemble includes:

a, b, c, f, g, h, and i
a. Metal overbed frame
b. Weights

c. Spreader

d. Knee sling

e. Kirschner wire

f. Rope

g. Pulleys

h. Adhesive straps

i. Elastic bandages

j. Razor

114 When Mr. Johnson arrives on the unit, the nurse talks with him and finds that he is 75 years old and weighs 150 pounds. The nurse prepares him for the application of traction by:

b and c

a. Painting his right leg with tincture of benzoin

b. Telling him what is going to be done

c. Washing and drying his right leg

d. Shaving the hair from his right leg

115 The nurse has included two spreaders in the equipment that has been brought to the bedside. What determines which one will be used?

c

a. The physician's preference

b. The size of the patient's knee

c. The size of the patient's ankle

116 Buck's extension traction was selected by the physician:

b and d

a. Since Mr. Johnson was too old for skeletal traction

b. To prevent muscle spasms

c. So that countertraction would not be needed

d. To relieve the pain

117 After the Buck's traction has been applied by the physician, the nurse periodically checks the patient for indications of _____

skin reaction; pressure sores; circulatory impairment; nerve damage; foot drop

_____ , _____ ,

_____ , _____

_____ , and _____ .

118 When checking Mr. Johnson, the nurse would observe:

All of these

a. His instep for signs of pressure

b. The skin color of his foot

c. His Achilles tendon for signs of pressure

d. His position in bed

119 When checking the patient, the nurse also looks at the traction equipment to check:

a, c, and d

a. The amount of weight in use

b. The position of the knee sling

c. The position of the spreader in relation to the pulley

d. The location of the weights

All of these

120 Since Mr. Johnson is 75 years old, which nursing problems should the nurse anticipate and plan for?

a. The formation of decubiti over bony prominences

b. Maintenance of adequate nutrition

c. Prevention of complications such as hypostatic pneumonia

d. Maintenance of good bowel function

adding a sling under the patient's knee

121 Later the physician tells the nurse that he would like to change Mr. Johnson's traction from Buck's extension to Russell's traction. This can be done by _____

_____ .

the knee sling for wrinkles

122 After Mr. Johnson's traction is changed to Russell's, changes must be made in his nursing care to include checking _____

_____ .

the instep; Achilles tendon; heels; posterior aspect of knee

123 The potential pressure points in Russell's traction are: _____ , _____ , _____ , and _____

_____ .

124 The nursing care plan for the patient in traction must be designed to meet the individual's needs. The patient's age, socio-economic background, length of hospitalization, and reason for being in traction must be considered when planning his care. Since the primary goal of orthopedic treatment is restoration of function, the nursing care plan should also focus on rehabilitation and the prevention of complications.

125 A 40-year-old woman, Miss Black, is admitted to the unit with arthritis of the neck. The physician requests that 10 pounds of inter-mittent cervical traction be applied. The traction is applied to (pro-

relieve pain

vide bed rest? relieve pain? reduce the fracture?).

encircling

126 Cervical traction is (balanced? skin? encircling?) traction.

127 When checking Miss Black, the nurse examined her chin and occipital areas:

a, b, and d

a. For signs of skin irritation

b. For indications of pressure sores

c. To see if the traction is effective

d. For indications of circulatory impairment

128 When checking the cervical traction equipment, the nurse verifies that:

a and d

a. The weights are hanging free
b. The spreader is against the pulley
c. The rope is on the bed
d. The traction is pulling in the desired direction

129 Miss Black has moved her body so that she is lying diagonally and the traction is no longer pulling in a straight line. The nurse should:

a and b

a. Change the patient's position
b. Explain to the patient the need for maintaining the proper alignment
c. Allow the patient to remain in the most comfortable position

130 Miss Black tells the nurse that her ears and chin are getting sore from being in traction. The nurse should:

a, b, and c

a. Remove the traction and examine the areas
b. Check the size of the spreader
c. Place padding inside the head halter to protect the areas
d. Remove 5 pounds of the weight so that the pressure isn't so great

skin, pelvic

131 Cervical traction is similar to (skeletal? skin? pelvic? balanced?) traction.

132 Complications that may occur in the use of skeletal traction

nerve damage; bone infection; pressure areas; circulatory impairment; deformities such as foot drop (any three, any order)

are: _____ , _____
_____ , and _____ .

133 List five pieces of equipment that are *essential* for applying skeletal traction without suspension.

a. Kirschner wire or Steinman pin or Kranendonk pin
b. U shaped spreader
c. Ropes
d. Pulleys
e. Weights

a. _____
b. _____
c. _____
d. _____
e. _____

equal to

opposite

will not

134 Countertraction is a pulling force (greater than? equal to?) and (in the same direction as? opposite?) the traction weight. If adequate countertraction is not provided, the traction (will? will not?) be effective.

135 Countertraction can be obtained for all traction methods by

tilting the bed in the opposite direction

_____
_____ .

136 When skeletal traction is in use and countertraction is obtained by using a Thomas splint, the fixed point that provides the opposing force is the _____.

ischial tuberosity

137 If the patient has a fractured right humerus and skeletal traction is applied by inserting a Kirschner wire in the proximal ulna, countertraction can be obtained by (elevating the foot of the bed on shock blocks? elevating the right side of the bed on shock blocks?).

elevating the right side of the bed on shock blocks

138 If the patient's right leg is suspended in a Thomas splint with a Pearson attachment, pressure areas may develop in the following locations: _____ , _____
_____ , _____
_____ , _____
_____ , and _____.

groin area; ischial tuberosity; posterior aspect of leg; Achilles tendon; all bony prominences

139 Which of the following are indications for the use of traction?
a. To provide rest for an inflamed joint
b. To reduce a fracture
c. To correct a deformity
d. To prevent complications
e. To provide muscle relaxation

a, b, c, and e

140 After being injured in an automobile accident, Mr. Brown is admitted to the orthopedic unit. His left leg is suspended in a Thomas splint with a Pearson attachment, and 20 pounds of weight have been attached to the Kirschner wire through his tibia. Since Mr. Brown's femur is fractured, the traction:
a. Must be uninterrupted
b. May be removed when union is complete
c. Must be continuous except when he is turned
d. Will reduce and immobilize the fracture

a, b, and d

141 Although the Kirschner wire may appear to be very painful, removal of the traction as an act of kindness could result in _____
_____.

painful muscle spasms and permanent injury to the patient (If fracture has been reduced, it could be pulled out of alignment.)

142 While assisting the physician in applying the traction, the nurse notes that the half ring of the Thomas splint is placed over the groin. Since the ring does not press against the ischial tuberosity, another means must be used to obtain _____.

countertraction

143 Later, Mr. Brown requests that the head of his bed be elevated. Which of the following statements is correct?
a. The head of his bed may be rolled up with no effect.

b

(The nurse should check with the physician when in doubt.)

b. Elevating the head of the bed may lessen the effect of the traction.

144 The factors that should be considered in the decision of whether or not to elevate the head of Mr. Brown's bed are: _____

_____

the prescribed direction of the pulling force; source of countertraction; type of traction apparatus; location of affected extremity

_____ , _____

_____ , _____

_____ , and _____

_____ .

145 As the traction was being applied, the physician placed Mr. Brown's left leg in an abducted position. The abduction (must? must not?) be maintained.

must

146 The signs of a bone infection at the site of a Kirschner wire are _____ , _____ , and _____ .

purulent drainage; foul odor
edema

147 Mr. Brown is reluctant to use the bedpan. Which nursing measures could be utilized?

a, b, and c

a. Reassure Mr. Brown that the traction will not be disturbed.
b. Obtain a fracture pan for Mr. Brown.
c. Teach Mr. Brown to use the overbed trapeze to aid in lifting onto the bedpan.
d. Explain to Mr. Brown that all traction patients have to use bedpans.

148 In addition to teaching Mr. Brown to use the overbed trapeze, the nurse could also teach him to _____

use the other leg to
assist in lifting

149 Since Mr. Brown will be immobilized in traction for approximately 2 months, his nursing care plan should include provisions for skin care to _____ .

prevent pressure areas

150 The nursing care of the traction patient includes frequent observations of both the _____ and the _____ .

patient; equipment

151 The nursing care of the traction patient focuses on the recognition of signs of complications such as _____

pressure areas; circulatory impairment; nerve damage; skin reaction

_____ , _____ , _____ , and _____ .

152 When the patient is to be placed in traction, the nurse (should? should not?) be responsible for the initial application of the weights.

should not

153 When countertraction is effective, the patient (does? does not?) have a tendency to slide toward the pulley.

does not

154 The methods of applying traction are _____, _____, _____, and _____.

manual
skin; skeletal; encircling

155 Match the method of applying traction with the appropriate time span descriptor.

Method	Time span descriptor
_____ 1. Skin	a. Emergency
_____ 2. Skeletal	b. Short-term
_____ 3. Manual	c. Long-term

b
c
a

156 Traction may be prescribed by the physician to _____ and/or _____ deformities.

prevent
correct

157 Traction is used in the treatment of fractures to _____ and/or _____ the fracture.

reduce
immobilize

158 When the patient has an inflamed joint, traction may be used to _____ the joint.

rest

159 Patients with low back pain are treated with traction in order to _____ by _____ .

flatten the lumbar curve
pulling on the lower back

160 The types of traction used in the treatment of low back pain include _____, _____, and _____ .

pelvic; 90-90 pelvic
Buck's extension

161 Traction immobilization of a fracture implies that the traction is to be _____ .

continuous

162 Briefly describe what occurs if the traction is removed from the fracture patient's extremity prematurely.

Fragment motion stimulates painful muscle spasms that can pull the fragments out of alignment and cause damage by severing a nerve or blood vessel.

163 Traction is used in the treatment of musculoskeletal injuries other than fractures to _____ _____ and to _____ _____ .

prevent and/or relieve muscle spasms; prevent or reduce edema

facilitate drainage

164 Traction may be prescribed in the treatment of infected wounds to _____ .

support the affected extremity; maintain the desired direction of the pulling force; maintain the desired degree of abduction

165 The patient's extremity may be placed in a Thomas splint with a Pearson attachment after surgery in order to _____ _____ , _____ _____ , and _____ _____ .

permits freedom of movement; facilitates nursing care

166 The advantages associated with the patient's being in balanced suspension are that it _____ _____ and _____ _____ .

True

False

True

False

167 Indicate whether the following statements are true or false:

_____a. The nurse plans the traction patient's care, incorporating his individual needs.

_____b. The nurse is responsible for the initial application of the traction weights.

_____c. The nursing care of the traction patient focuses on observing the patient for signs and symptoms of complications.

_____d. Care of the traction patient is primarily focused on the traction equipment.

Traction is the application of a pulling force.

168 Define traction.

to restore function to the injured part

169 The goal of orthopedic treatment is _____ _____ .

Ask your instructor to review and/or discuss your list in class to identify how the text did or did not help you solve the problems or answer your questions.

170 On a separate piece of paper list the nursing care problems and questions that you have identified when giving care to a traction patient.

CHAPTER 8

Principles of nursing care of the patient in a cast

1 Numerous technological innovations are occurring in orthopedics. Whereas in the past edition this chapter was limited to a discussion of plaster casts, it now contains information about three types of cast materials. Although the cast materials differ, the principles of nursing care are very much the same for all three types. The materials used to apply a cast are plaster of paris, fiberglass, and thermolabile plastic. The cast materials differ; the principles of nursing care (remain the same? differ greatly?).

remain the same

2 The types of cast materials are _____ _____ , _____ , and _____

plaster of paris; fiberglass; thermolabile plastic

_____ .

3 Thermolabile plastic, under trade names such as Orthoplast, can be molded to fit an extremity and/or the torso after being heated in warm water. Once the material is warm, it will adhere to itself. The term thermolabile implies that the material can be molded after a change in _____ .

temperature

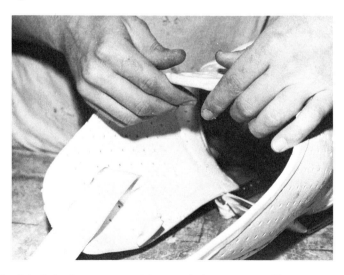

Fig. 8-1. Orthoplast cast material comes in large squares. The squares are cut and, after being heated, are molded to fit the body part to be casted. (Courtesy Johnson & Johnson, New Brunswick, N.J.)

4 The type of cast material that is moldable after heating is

_____ .

5 The fiberglass cast is formed from rolls of fiberglass tape that have been impregnated with a photosensitive resin that requires processing under an ultraviolet light to harden. In order to set the cast, the thermolabile material must be _____ and the fiberglass must be treated with _____ _____ .

6 After being cured under the ultraviolet light, the fiberglass cast is lightweight yet very hard. The fiberglass cast is a fiberglass tape which contains a _____ .

7 A plaster cast is a bandage that has been impregnated with anhydrous gypsum, moistened, and molded around an area of the body. It then sets quickly, forming a cement-like substance. The chemical that is the active ingredient in a plaster bandage is _____ _____ .

8 The types of cast materials used in modern orthopedics include _____ , _____ , and _____ .

9 Casts are used in the treatment of many orthopedic conditions for the purpose of immobilizing the affected part. Immobilization may be necessary to maintain the position of fracture fragments; to restrict usage of or support diseased or weakened bones, joints, or muscles; and to prevent or correct deformities. The primary reason for applying a plaster cast is to _____ the affected part.

10 The physician frequently applies a cast to the affected extremity after a closed reduction. Why would a cast be applied after a closed reduction?

11 The physician applies a body cast to a young girl with severe lordosis. The cast is being used to _____ _____ .

12 Mr. Brown has had a tumor removed from his left femur. At the same time a portion of the femur was excised. After surgery the physician applied a cast in order to _____

support the weakened
bone

_____ or _____

_____ .

13 Immobilization of the affected body part by the application of a cast may be selected as the treatment modality in order to:

a, b, and d

a. Prevent a fracture
b. Prevent a deformity
c. Prevent ambulation
d. Permit a joint to heal

14 The nurse should prepare the patient for the application of a cast by talking with him about what will be done and what will occur afterward. The nurse might tell the patient that a cast is being applied

immobilize
(Interpret word so patient understands.)

to _____ the affected part.

15 In order to more fully inform the patient, the nurse must know what materials are likely to be used, what parts of the body will be included in the cast, and how the cast will be applied. The type of material used dictates what procedures will be followed in the application process and the nursing care of the patient afterward. Therefore, an overview of the application process follows.

16 In some institutions, there is a special "cast" or "plaster" room or an equipment cart that contains all the necessary supplies for the application of a cast. Many times there is a nursing attendant or orthopedic technician assigned to the room who prepares all the equipment and assists the physician. The nurse needs to be familiar with the equipment and steps of application to be able to assist. In

prepare the patient

addition to preparing the equipment, the nurse should _____

_____ .

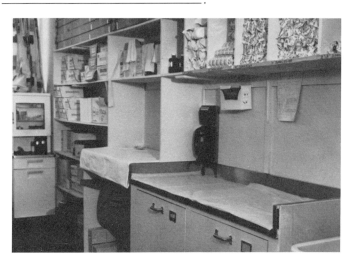

Fig. 8-2. Supplies needed for the application of a plaster cast, stored in the plaster room at The Ohio State University Hospitals, Columbus, Ohio.

17 Regardless of the type of material used, the cast application procedure is performed in essentially the same manner by all physicians although there are minor variations. As a first step, a cotton stockinette is placed over the area or extremity to which the plaster is to be applied. This step is omitted in the application of thermolabile plastic. The stockinette used for the fiberglass cast is a specially treated material. The stockinette protects the patient's skin and provides a first layer of padding. Padding is needed since the plaster bandage, after it sets, forms a (gypsumate? soft? cement-like?) substance.

cement-like

18 A cast must be applied so that it fits the affected part snugly in order to achieve the goal of immobilization. The area or extremity within the cast will be in contact with the firm surface, thereby creating a potential for the development of complications. Thus it is absolutely essential that the stockinette and other padding be smooth, since wrinkles or ridges in it could contribute to the development of pressure sores, or could cause nerve damage or circulatory

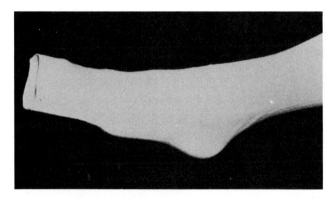

Fig. 8-3. Ankle with stockinette applied.

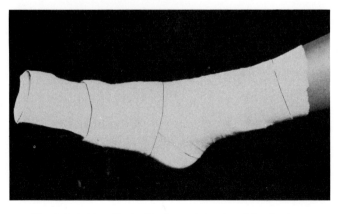

Fig. 8-4. Ankle with stockinette and sheet wadding in place.

impairment. Three complications associated with casts are

pressure sores; nerve
damage; circulatory
impairment

_____ , _____ .

and _____ .

19 When a plaster cast is applied, sheet wadding is wrapped around the area or extremity covered by stockinette, and pieces of felt padding are placed over bony prominences. Like stockinette, sheet wadding and felt padding are applied primarily to (keep the area dry? provide comfort for the patient? prevent pressure sores?).

prevent pressure sores

20 These three layers not only protect the area or extremity but also form a foundation for the plaster cast. A plaster cast is being applied to the patient's ankle. How is the extremity protected?

By placing stockinette and
sheet wadding over the
entire area and padding the
malleoli with felt.

21 Commercially prepared plaster bandages come packaged in rolls. After the package is removed, the roll is placed *vertically* in a bucket of tepid water. When the plaster bandages are placed in water, bubbles rise from them as the anhydrous gypsum absorbs water. When the bubbling stops, the bandages are ready for immediate use. The plaster bandages are prepared for use by:

b, d, and e

a. Shaking away the loose gypsum
b. Removing the package

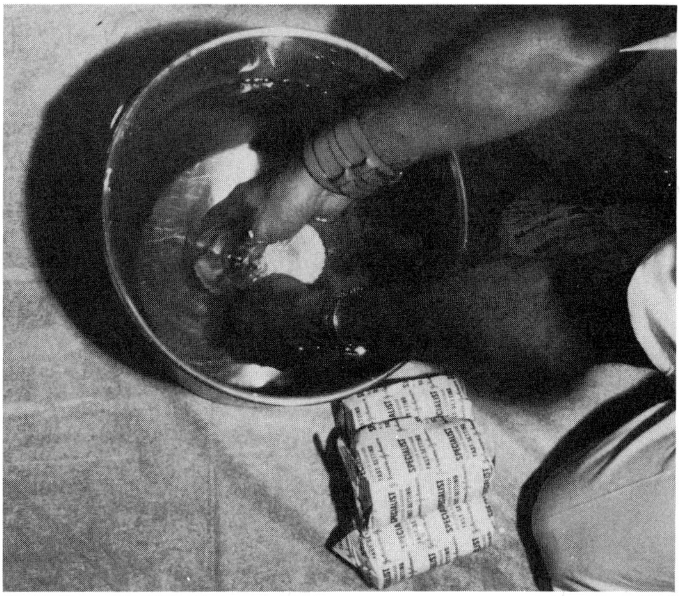

Fig. 8-5. Plaster roll is placed vertically in bucket of tepid water. Note bubbles rising from plaster roll.

c. Placing them in a bucket of water

d. Placing them in a bucket of tepid water

e. Standing them on end in the water

22 The physician determines the size and type of cast, in what position the affected part is to be immobilized and maintained, and the type of cast material to be used. One general principle that the physician follows is that if the extremity is fractured, the joint above and the joint below the fracture site are included in the cast. Mrs. Smith has fallen and broken her tibia. Briefly describe the cast to be applied.

The cast must include the ankle and knee joints.

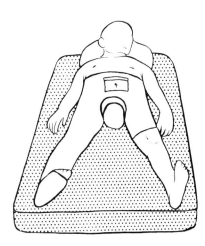

Fig. 8-6. Spica cast that includes the knee and hip of the affected side and the contralateral hip.

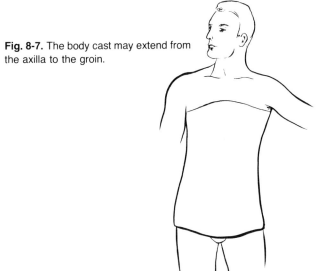

Fig. 8-7. The body cast may extend from the axilla to the groin.

23 With the newer cast materials this principle is not always followed. The type of cast is determined not only by the fracture site but also on the basis of the physician's treatment approach. The type of cast also depends on the underlying rationale for immobilization. The reasons for using a cast to immobilize an extremity and/or the body include:

a. _____

_____

b. _____

_____

c. _____

_____

a. To maintain fracture fragment position

b. To restrict usage of or support diseased or weakened bones, joints, or muscles

c. To prevent or correct deformities

24 A nurse or other assistant may be needed to support the affected limb while the physician applies the padding and plaster. When a plaster cast is being applied to prevent or correct a deformity and the physician places the extremity in a specified position, the nurse

b, c, and d

a. Adjusts the position as requested by the patient
b. Adjusts the position as requested by the physician
c. Maintains the indicated degree of abduction
d. Maintains the indicated degree of internal rotation

25 The physician, wearing gloves to protect the hands, carefully molds the plaster to conform to the patient's muscular and bony contours. The wet plaster must be handled with the palms of the hands because the fingers could make indentations on the outer surface. These indentations would become bumps on the inner surface of the cast. As with the stockinette, any bumps inside the cast could

pressure sores; nerve damage; circulatory impairment

cause _____ , _____

_____ , or _____ .

26 Until the plaster is firm, the enclosed limb must remain immobile since any joint movement might cause wrinkles or ridges within the cast. The nurse is responsible for supporting the patient's ex-

immobile

designated position

tremity as the cast is being applied in order to keep it _____ and to maintain the _____ .

27 When the patient is having a plaster cast applied, the nurse is re-

preparing the patient

preparing the equipment

holding the affected part

sponsible for _____ ,

_____ ,

and _____ .

28 The physician may incorporate a walking heel into a cast being applied to a lower limb if the patient will be allowed to bear weight

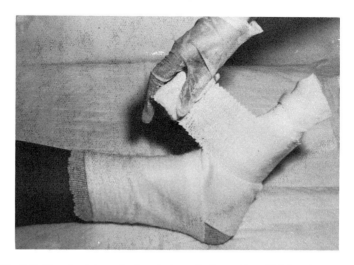

Fig. 8-8. The physician rolls the plaster onto the ankle, which has been prepared with stockinette and sheet wadding.

on the extremity. The equipment that should be prepared for the application of a walking cast (plaster) includes: _____, _____ , _____ , _____ , _____ , _____ , and _____ .

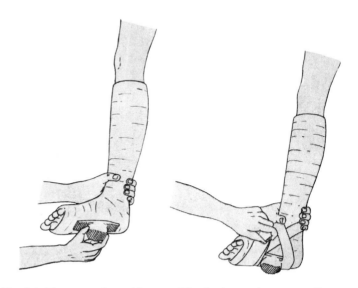

Fig. 8-9. The steps of attaching a walking heel to a plaster cast. (Courtesy Zimmer · USA, Warsaw, Ind.)

stockinette; sheet wadding; felt padding; walking heel; plaster bandages; bucket of water; gloves

29 If the plaster cast needs to be supported during the application, the palm of the hand should be used; the fingers could _____ _____ _____ .

mold the cast and result in bumps on the inner surface of the cast

30 When preparing to apply a thermolabile plastic cast, the physician measures the area to be covered and makes a paper pattern or template. After checking that the pattern fits the patient, the physician then uses the pattern to cut what is needed from a large piece of the plastic. The application of the plastic cast is different from the application of a plaster cast in that no _____ , _____ , or _____ are used.

stockinette

sheet wadding; felt pads

31 The cut piece of plastic is heated in hot water and then molded to the patient's body or extremity. The overlapped edges of the plastic adhere to one another, so no bandage or adhesive is necessary. The casting procedure is complete when the plastic is cool and hard. When a thermolabile cast is applied, the size of the piece to be used is determined by the physician, who measures the patient and makes

pattern or template

a _____ .

32 Polypropylene stockinette that sheds water is used as the base layer of the fiberglass cast. A special web wrap of polypropylene padding is used to provide additional cushioning for bony prominences and pressure points just as is done with the plaster cast. Fiber-

stockinette

glass and plaster casts are alike in that _____

padding

and _____ are used.

33 The fiberglass cast is molded to the patient's muscular and bony contours in steps similar to those used in applying a plaster cast. However, the physician must use a special silicone hand cream to facilitate smoothing and blending the layers of impregnated fiberglass tape. The silicone cream also protects the physician's hands. The applications of a plaster cast and a fiberglass cast are similar because:

b, c, d, and e

a. Both use materials affected by temperature.

b. The physician's hands are protected while working.

c. Bony prominences are padded in both.

d. The layer next to the skin is stockinette.

e. Both require molding of the cast during application.

f. Both are self-adhering substances.

34 After the fiberglass cast is molded to the physician's specifications, the body part with the cast on it is placed under an ultraviolet light for several minutes to cure or set. Molding of the fiberglass cast

silicone cream

requires smoothing and blending of the tape layers with _____
_____ .

35 Since care is taken during the application of a fiberglass cast to mold the cast and pad bony prominences, the nurse may anticipate the possibility of the same complications as may occur with a plaster

pressure sores; nerve
damage; circulatory
impairment

cast. These complications include _____
_____ , _____ , and _____
_____ .

36 All three types of casts are radiolucent—that is, in order for

can remain in place

x-rays to be taken the cast (must be removed? can remain in place?).

37 The affected extremity is held in the position specified by the physician to:

c and d

a. Prevent pain

b. Prevent pressure areas

c. Immobilize the fracture reduction

d. Maintain the deformity correction

38 As each layer of plaster is applied, the cast sets and must be supported so that it does not crack. The cast should be supported by (both hands? the fingertips? a sling? the palm of the hand?).

39 When the application of the plaster cast is complete, the physician may trim the edges of the cast with plaster shears or a plaster knife, or the final trimming may be done after the cast is dry. Which supplies are used in the application of a plaster cast to the arm?

a, b, c, d, f, h, i, and j
*(Sling and Ace bandages may
be put on later but are not
needed to apply the plaster
cast.)*

a. Rubber gloves   g. Ace bandages
b. Plaster knife   h. Plaster bandages
c. Felt padding   i. Water
d. Sheet wadding   j. Plaster shears
e. Walking heel   k. Sling
f. Stockinette   l. Silicone cream

40 When the application is completed, the plaster should be washed from the exposed part of the extremity. This allows the nurse to observe the fingers and toes for signs of _____ _____.

41 Thermolabile plastic and fiberglass casts are hard within a few minutes of application, while a plaster cast takes much longer to harden. The rapidity of time required for a hard cast is one of the primary advantages of the thermolabile and fiberglass casts. However, the need to process the fiberglass cast under an ultraviolet light is viewed as a disadvantage since it may be difficult to maintain the desired position of the extremity during this step. One basic difference between the new cast materials and plaster of paris is

_____ _____.

42 As the plaster begins to set, the patient will begin to feel warmth from the chemical process. The feeling of warmth will continue until the cast is completely dry. When preparing the patient for the application of a plaster cast, the nurse (should? should not?) tell him to expect the feeling of warmth.

43 Until the cast is completely dry, the patient should not be permitted to place the cast on a hard, flat surface. If a body or spica cast has been applied, the patient should be placed on a (soft? firm? hard?) bed.

44 Pillows should be used to support the curves of a cast. If a damp cast is not supported, it will lose its shape and be ineffective, or it may put pressure on the tissues beneath it. Which of the following is (are) true?

a. Improper handling of a wet cast can lead to the development of complications.
b. Improper handling of a damp cast may result in an ineffective cast.
c. Joint motion during application of the cast is permitted.
d. Proper support of a damp plaster cast is not essential to maintain its shape and size.

45 A plaster cast requires approximately 48 hours to dry completely. To promote drying, the cast should be uncovered and exposed to the air. The damp cast should be supported by:

a. Firm bed
b. Sandbags
c. Pillows
d. Rolled sheets

46 If an external heat source is used to dry the cast, it must be used carefully because the heat from the drying process may burn the patient. The time needed for the plaster cast to dry completely is (20 to 24? 36? 46 to 50? 72?) hours.

47 When the plaster cast is dry it will be hard, white, shiny, and odorless. Use of an external heat source is hazardous because the heat from the drying process may (dry the cast too fast? burn the patient? make the cast too hard?).

48 The patient in a cast must be turned every 4 to 6 hours so that the cast will dry evenly and thoroughly. The completely dry cast is (firm? white? shiny? hard? smooth? odorless?).

49 The major advantage of the thermolabile plastic and the fiberglass cast is that _____.

50 One major disadvantage of the fiberglass cast is that _____ _____.

51 Two disadvantages of the thermolabile plastic cast are that _____, and _____ _____.

52 The nursing care of the patient in a cast should include frequent observations for signs of complications. Early recognition of the signs of complications is essential, since prolonged pressure or impairment of circulation could result in extensive and/or permanent damage. The nurse should promptly report signs or symptoms of complications because the complications may lead to

_____ and/or _____

damage.

53 These complications are manifested by edema, pain, changes in skin color and temperature, and decreased digit mobility and sensation. A thorough assessment of the patient to obtain measurements on these variables must be done before the cast is applied. It is essential that the nurse making the initial assessment record her observations and measurements so that they are available for comparison with post–cast application data. The recording of the initial assessment should include the following observations:

a. The absence or presence of _____ or _____

b. If present, the location of _____ and _____

c. A description of the skin _____ and _____

d. Patient's ability to _____ and _____ digits

54 The clinical signs are not uniquely related to each of the complications; that is, the signs of nerve damage, circulatory impairment, and pressure area development overlap. For example, pain or numbness may be present in both nerve damage and pressure sores. Therefore, when indications of complications are observed, they should be promptly reported to the physician. Two reportable observations

are _____ and _____ .

55 To observe the patient for signs of circulatory impairment, check the color of the skin of the toes or fingers of the affected extremity. The skin color of the toes or fingers of the affected extremity should be pink. If they are cyanotic or pale, they should be further checked by doing the blanching test. When checking for indications of circu-

latory impairment, the nurse should first check _____

_____ .

56 The blanching test is easily performed by pressing on a toenail or fingernail of the affected limb. With pressure, the nail turns white; when the pressure is released it should immediately turn pink. The

blanching test should be done if the toes or fingers are _____

or _____ .

57 At the same time, the nurse should also check the temperature of the skin of the toes or fingers. The skin should be warm. In the

blanching test, the nail turns _____ , then _____ .

58 If the patient was able to move his fingers or toes before the cast was applied, he should be able to move them afterward. The nurse color

temperature

should ask him to move them while checking the skin _____ and skin _____ .

59 In addition to checking the mobility of the patient's fingers or toes, the nurse should also check the amount of swelling. The nurse should check the fingers or toes of the affected limb to make certain that all signs are normal. Normal responses are:

a. Pink
b. Warm
c. Patient able to move
   fingers or toes

a. Skin color— _____
b. Skin temperature— _____
c. Mobility— _____

60 Pulselessness is the ultimate indication of circulatory impairment; however, the locations where a pulse might be felt are often covered by the cast. Therefore, the nurse must rely on other indications of circulatory impairment. The patient's right arm is in a cast. The nurse checks his fingers and sees that they are cyanotic. The nurse would then do the _____ .

blanching test

61 Pain and numbness are also indications of impaired circulation. Which of the following are *not* indicative of impaired circulation?

b and f

a. Increased swelling
b. Pink skin color
c. Cyanotic fingers or toes
d. Loss of motion
e. Pale fingers or toes
f. Ability to move fingers or toes
g. Cold fingers or toes

62 The circulation to the patient's fingers or toes may be constricted by swelling of the affected extremity within the cast (compartment syndrome). To prevent or reduce edema, the affected extremity may be elevated, icebags may be placed next to the cast, and the patient should be encouraged to move his fingers or toes. The presence of continued edema requires action; the physician must decide whether the cast should be adjusted. The patient has a cast on his right ankle and his toes are edematous; the swelling can be reduced by (extremity elevation? cast removal? ice application? digital motion?).

extremity elevation, ice
application, digital motion

63 The physician usually prefers to split or bivalve the plaster or fiberglass cast to restore circulation rather than to remove it entirely. Impaired circulation is considered an emergency because if not promptly treated it could result in (an occluded artery? necrosis of the tissues? deformity? occlusion of a vein?).

necrosis of the tissues,
deformity
(The circulation is impaired
because the vessels are occluded. Review discussion
of compartment syndrome.)

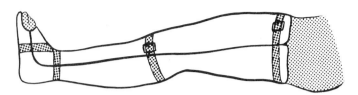

Fig. 8-10. This long leg cast has been bivalved, and the anterior and posterior portions are held in place by straps so that the leg remains immobilized.

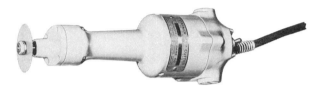

Fig. 8-11. An electric cast cutter. (Courtesy Zimmer · USA, Warsaw, Ind.)

64 The cast cutter should be kept readily available on the nursing unit for such an emergency. To bivalve a cast is to (split? remove?) it.

split

65 After the physician has bivalved the cast, the affected extremity should be elevated until the edema decreases and adequate circulation is reestablished. The patient has a cast on his right ankle and his toes are edematous. The swelling can be treated by:

a. Elevating the extremity
b. Placing icebags next to the cast
c. Having patient move his toes
d. Bivalving the cast

a. _____
b. _____
c. _____
d. _____

66 After the cast has been on for several days, the possibility of circulatory impairment and nerve damage from the cast decreases. However, pressure areas may develop over an extended period of time. Complaints of itching or burning pain are indications of a pressure sore and should never be ignored. Two signs of pressure area development are _____ and _____ .

burning pain; itching

67 The development of a pressure sore is not always preceded by this sign and may not be detected. An untreated pressure area eventually becomes an open draining wound. Therefore, the patient's cast should be inspected each day since indications of a pressure sore, such as an unpleasant odor from the cast, drainage from under or through the cast, or a warm area on the cast, might otherwise be overlooked. The signs of a pressure sore under a plaster cast are:

a. Burning pain
b. Itching
c. Drainage
d. Unpleasant odor from cast
e. Warm area on cast

a. _____

b. _____

c. _____

d. _____

e. _____

68 After the initial swelling has subsided, edema of the fingers and toes or an elevated body temperature is also an indication of the presence of a pressure area. As the nurse cares for the patient in a cast she is alert for signs of a pressure area forming beneath the cast. Match the sign with the sense used by the nurse.

	Sign	Sense used
c	_____ 1. Drainage from under the cast	a. Touch
a or c	_____ 2. Swelling of fingers or toes	b. Smell
a	_____ 3. Warm area on cast	c. Sight
a	_____ 4. Elevated body temperature	d. Hearing
b	_____ 5. Foul odor from the cast	
d	_____ 6. Patient's complaint of itching under the cast	

69 Which of the following are *not* indications of a pressure sore on the patient's heel when he has a cast on the ankle and lower leg?

b and e

a. Patient's body temperature is 102° F.
b. Patient is complaining of pain in ankle.
c. The cast has an odor of purulent discharge.
d. The cast has bloody drainage on it in the heel area.
e. The patient's toes are normal size.

70 The physician must be notified of any indications of a forming pressure area under a cast. The nurse would report which of the following:

101° F.
present
present
foul
itching

a. Body temperature: (99.2°F.? 101°F.?)
b. Swelling of fingers: (absent? present?)
c. Drainage from cast: (absent? present?)
d. Odor from cast: (foul? none?)
e. Patient complaints: (pressure? itching?)

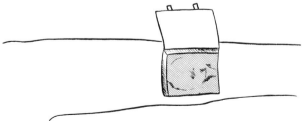

Fig. 8-12. Plaster cast with window cut over knee area.

111

71 When the patient has a plaster cast, the physician will usually cut out and remove a square section (window) of the cast over the suspected pressure sore. The physician can then inspect the wound and treat it through the window.

72 While the square portion (window) is out of the cast, the physician may check it for ridges and wrinkles that might have been the source of the pressure. After treating the pressure sore, the physician will insert padding to apply pressure and prevent edema, then tape the square back in place. The window is removed from the cast so that the physician may _____ and _____ the pressure area.

inspect; treat

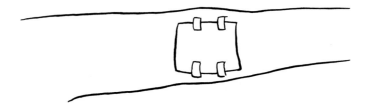

Fig. 8-13. The cast window is taped back in place after inspection and treatment of the area.

73 If the patient in a body or spica cast complains of vomiting, constipation, or abdominal pain or distention, it should be reported to the physician. Constriction of the abdomen by the cast may cause a paralytic ileus. The possible complications from a plaster cast are

nerve damage; circulatory impairment (compartment syndrome); pressure sores; paralytic ileus

_____ , _____ _____ , _____ , and _____ .

74 The initial treatment of a paralytic ileus may include cutting a window in the cast over the abdominal area. The indications of a paralytic ileus include patient complaints of:

a. Vomiting
b. Constipation
c. Abdominal pain
d. Abdominal distention

a. _____
b. _____
c. _____
d. _____

75 The patient in a spica or body cast should also be observed for signs of respiratory distress. Occasionally the cast is too tight and restricts expansion of the lungs; other times the patient is unable to adjust to the cast and reacts by hyperventilating. The patient in a spica cast must be observed for which of the following?

b, c, d, and e

a. Diarrhea   d. Digital cyanosis
b. Dyspnea   e. Drainage
c. Distension

76 Associate the following complications with the appropriate approach:

c, d   _____ 1. Circulatory impairment   a. Patient reassurance

a   _____ 2. Respiratory distress   b. Window cast

b   _____ 3. Paralytic ileus   c. Elevate extremity

b, d   _____ 4. Pressure area   d. Bivalve cast

77 List the basic nursing actions performed in the care of the patient before and after the application of a cast.

a. Make initial assessment

b. Prepare patient

c. Prepare equipment and supplies

d. Assist physician

e. Support extremity during application

f. Observe for indications of complications

g. Report indications of complications

h. Assist in treatment of complications

a. _____

b. _____

c. _____

d. _____

e. _____

f. _____

g. _____

h. _____

78 Three people will be needed to turn the patient in a damp (plaster) spica or large body cast. After the cast is dry, two nurses, or possibly only one, will be needed if the patient is able to assist. Before turning the patient, the nurse should check the toes of the affected leg for _____ , _____

skin color; skin temperature; mobility; swelling

_____ , _____ , and _____ .

79 When the patient is in a spica cast, he should be turned on the leg not in the cast. If both legs are included in the cast, the patient should be turned on the unoperated side. (Review Chapter 2.)

80 The first step of turning is to pull the patient to the side of the bed. Would you move the patient in Fig. 8-14 toward _A_ or _B?_

toward A   _____

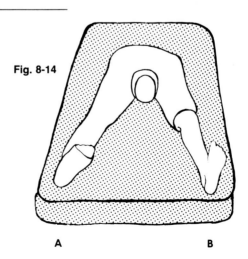

Fig. 8-14

A   B

81 The damp plaster cast must be supported as the patient is turned to keep it from cracking. Pillows must be placed on the bed to support the cast and the patient's extremities, regardless of the type of cast. What part of the hands does the nurse use to support the plaster cast? _____

the palms

82 To prepare for turning, the patient should place his arms either over his head or at his sides. The patient is then gently rolled over. The nurse on the opposite side of the bed slowly eases him onto the waiting pillows. The curves of the damp plaster cast are supported on pillow because _____ _____ _____.

it could lose (change) its shape and become in-effective or cause pressure areas

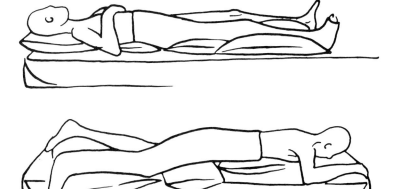

Fig. 8-15. Pillows are used to support the spica cast in the supine and prone positions.

83 The abduction bar of a spica cast is intended to maintain the abduction; it should not be used as a handle to lift or turn the patient. Number the steps of turning the patient in a spica cast in the order of their occurrence.

3 _____ Place pillows on bed to receive patient.
4 _____ Have patient move arms over head.
1 _____ Decide which direction to turn patient.
5 _____ Roll patient over.
2 _____ Move patient to side of bed.

84 The patient must be instructed to place only his fingers inside his cast. Foreign objects can become wedged under the cast and cause pressure sores. Pointed objects used for scratching may puncture the skin and be a source of infection. The patient complains of occasional itching inside his cast. What may he use to scratch the area? _____

his fingers

114

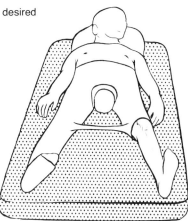

Fig. 8-16. The bar between the knees maintains the desired degree of abduction.

85 The patient is taught not to put objects inside his cast because:

a, b, and d

a. A coathanger used for scratching could puncture the skin.
b. A pill hidden from the nurse could cause a pressure area.
c. A towel left in place after the bath could cause swelling.
d. A lead pencil used for scratching could cause an infection.

86 The cast may not fit the extremity snugly at the edges; the nurse or patient can thus insert his or her fingers under the edge of the cast. As much of the skin under the cast as can be reached by the patient or nurse must be washed each day. After being washed and dried, the skin near the edge of the cast should be checked for signs of rubbing or irritation. Lotion or rubbing alcohol can be applied to the skin near the edge and under the cast. The skin near the edge of the

rubbing

irritation

cast should be checked for signs of _____ and

_____ .

87 A plaster cast must be protected from moisture and soiling because it becomes limp and ineffective when wet and retains the odor when soiled. The thermolabile and fiberglass casts can be washed without harm and do not retain odors. Two occasions when care must be exercised to prevent a body or spica cast from moisture are

taking a bath; using
the bedpan

when the patient is _____ or _____

_____ .

88 Thermolabile and fiberglass casts do not present as many problems since they are both waterproof. It is possible to shower or bathe without harming these casts. However, it is difficult to dry the skin under these casts, so they are not routinely immersed; care must be taken to prevent urine or feces from getting under these casts. When

weakened

is not

wet, the plaster cast is (weakened? hardened?) and the fiberglass cast (is? is not?) harmed.

89 The posterior edges of a plaster spica cast must be protected

115

when the patient is using the bedpan. Any type of waterproof material can be used by cutting it to fit the posterior edges. Just before the patient gets on the bedpan, the waterproof material can be powdered, slipped under the edge of the cast, and turned back. The cast is protected because:

a, b, and d

a. It becomes limp when wet
b. It retains the odor if soiled with urine or feces
c. It looks bad if wet
d. It becomes ineffective when wet

90 The patient must then be assisted onto the bedpan. This can be done either by lifting the patient straight up or by rolling the patient on his side and then back onto the bedpan. The posterior edge of the cast can be protected by using (plastic sheeting? waxed paper? oilcloth? plastic food wrap?).

plastic sheeting,
oilcloth, plastic food wrap
(all are waterproof)

91 A fracture pan is often more comfortable and easier for the patient to use than a regular bedpan. After the patient has finished using the bedpan, the waterproof material should be removed and either cleaned or discarded. The waterproof material will slip under the edge of the cast more readily if it is _____ .

powdered

92 If possible, the female patient should be taught to use a female urinal, since it is more comfortable to use than a bedpan. Waterproof material is used:

b

a. To make the use of the bedpan more comfortable
b. To protect the cast from moisture
c. To make it easier for the patient to get on the bedpan

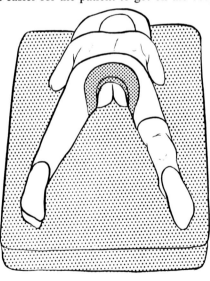

Fig. 8-17. The shaded area represents waterproof material that has been inserted to protect the posterior edge of the cast.

93 Other phases of hygiene should be continued, with the patient doing as much of his own care as possible. The patient in a spica cast should be able to:

a, b, d, and e
(He can't reach his feet.)

a. Wash the upper part of his body
b. Brush his own teeth
c. Wash his feet
d. Comb his hair
e. Clean his fingernails

94 Unless he has a medical condition that contraindicates it, a regular diet is prescribed for the orthopedic patient. A low-calorie diet may be prescribed for the patient in a body or spica cast who might gain weight because of his inactivity. A nursing care measure that promotes digestion would be to elevate the head of the bed while the patient is eating. True or false?

True
(Review Chapter 2
if necessary.)

95 In addition to using the extremities not included in the cast for hygienic measures, the patient should also utilize them for other activities to maintain their function and to prevent disuse atrophy of the muscles, joint stiffness, and osteoporosis. List the complications associated with use of a plaster cast.

a. Circulatory impairment
b. Nerve damage
c. Pressure sores
d. Paralytic ileus
e. Respiratory distress
f. Muscle atrophy
g. Joint stiffness
h. Osteoporosis
(see Chapter 14)

a. _____
b. _____
c. _____
d. _____
e. _____
f. _____
g. _____
h. _____

96 With the physician's approval, the patient may perform isometric exercises with the muscles included within the cast. For example, a patient in a spica or leg cast could do quadriceps-setting exercises. Doing isometric exercises will help to prevent _____ _____ and muscle _____ _____ .

osteoporosis
disuse atrophy

97 The patient who has a cast on his leg must strengthen his arms so that he will be able to walk with crutches when the physician permits him to. The patient could:

All of these

a. Do as much of his own bath as possible
b. Do arm exercises
c. Lift weights
d. Assist in moving himself

98 The nursing care plan of the patient in a cast should focus on:

a. Maintaining the use of the unaffected extremities
b. Limiting the patient's activities
c. Assisting the patient to care for himself
d. Early recognition of signs of complications

99 After the physician has removed the cast, the affected extremity will be weak and will require support. The patient has just had the

cast removed from his leg. The patient (can? cannot?) walk on that leg because it is (strong? weak?).

100 Which part of Fig. 8-18 shows the proper way to support the

leg? _____

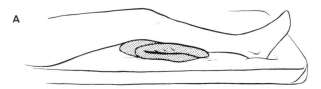

A

Fig. 8-18

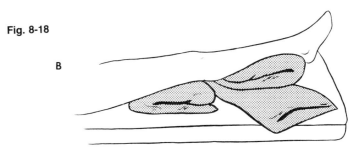

B

101 The skin that has been under the cast will be very dry and flaky. The layers of dead skin must be soaked off gradually. The layers of dead skin may also be softened with oil. Forcible removal of the dead skin can cause open wounds. Which of the following can be used to remove the dead skin from an extremity after a plaster cast has been removed?

a. Soaking in warm water
b. Washing with soap and water using a brush
c. Soaking in soapy water
d. Applying liberal amounts of mineral oil

102 Mrs. Smith fell on the ice this morning on the way to the Senior Citizens' Center. The physician has reduced the fracture and applied a plaster cast to her right wrist as pictured in Fig. 8-19. Mrs. Smith has been admitted to the orthopedic unit. The initial assessment of Mrs. Smith should include some observations about her

fingers (right hand): _____ , _____

_____ , _____ ,

and _____ .

103 The nurse notes that Mrs. Smith's cast is still very damp. The nurse:

c

a. Has the patient rest the cast on the overbed table
b. Covers the entire right arm with a blanket
c. Supports the cast with a pillow

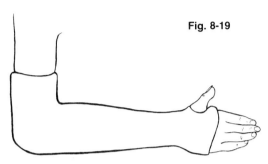

Fig. 8-19

104 An hour later, the nurse notices that Mrs. Smith's fingers (right hand) are puffy. She tells Mrs. Smith to:

c

a. Move the fingers once in a while, but not if they hurt
b. Hold her fingers in a flexed position
c. Move her fingers as much as possible
d. Keep her fingers covered

105 Since Mrs. Smith's fingers (right hand) are pale, the nurse

circulation; impaired

suspects that the _____ is _____ .

106 One way the nurse could check Mrs. Smith's circulation would

blanching test

be by doing the _____ .

107 If the circulation is impaired, Mrs. Smith might complain of

pain; numbness

_____ or _____ .

108 Which of the following nursing care measures would help reduce the edema in Mrs. Smith's fingers?

c and e

a. Elevating the head of the bed
b. Applying an icebag to the fingers
c. Elevating the entire right arm on two pillows
d. Applying an icebag to the elbow
e. Placing icebags alongside the cast

109 Thirty minutes after taking these nursing measures, the nurse checks Mrs. Smith again for signs of *impaired circulation*. After checking the nurse notifies the physician because:

pale or cyanotic

a. The fingers are _____ in color.

cool

b. The skin temperature is _____ .

has not

c. The swelling (has? has not?) decreased.

cannot

d. The patient (can? cannot?) move her fingers.

110 When the physician arrives on the unit, the nurse has the equipment ready, including the _____.

111 Usually the physician does not remove the cast but does _____ it.

112 After the swelling goes down, Mrs. Smith progresses nicely and is to be discharged. Her family should be taught:
a. To do as much as possible for Mrs. Smith
b. The signs of a pressure area
c. To have Mrs. Smith dangle her arm at her side as much as possible
d. To keep the cast clean and dry

113 If Mrs. Smith's cast had been fiberglass rather than plaster, the nurse would have changed the nursing care by:
a. Not observing for circulatory impairment
b. Not using icebags to reduce edema
c. Not exercising care to keep the cast dry
d. Not being concerned about the cast being dry

114 Mr. Jones was taken to surgery for incision and drainage of an abscess on his right distal tibia. When returned from surgery, he had a cast on (from his right knee to his toes). The plaster cast was applied to:
a. Immobilize the fracture
b. Provide rest and support for the bone
c. Prevent deformity
d. Correct a deformity

115 Mr. Jones is very willing to do as much for himself as possible. His nursing care plan should include:
a. Teaching him arm exercises
b. Encouraging him to lift himself with the trapeze
c. Teaching him about putting only his fingers into his cast
d. Encouraging him to eat a well-balanced diet

116 Two weeks after surgery, Mr. Jones complains of itching and a burning pain in his right heel. The complaints should be reported to the physician because _____
_____.

117 The nurse would check Mr. Jones' cast for other signs of a pressure area, including:

a. Firmness	d. Foreign objects
b. Discharge or drainage	e. Warm area over heel
c. Foul odor	

118 What equipment should the nurse have available for the physician after reporting observations?

a, b, e, and f

a. Dressings   d. Walking heel
b. Adhesive tape   e. Plaster shears
c. Bucket of water   f. Cast cutter

119 The equipment is necessary because the physician probably will (remove? repair? cut a window in?) the cast.

cut a window in

120 After cutting a window in the cast, the physician will:

b and d

a. Discard the square of plaster
b. Examine the area
c. Have the nurse discard the square of plaster
d. Treat the wound

121 The physician applies a dressing and leaves orders for it to be changed every 4 hours. The nurse:

a, b, and d

a. Applies a fresh dressing as ordered
b. Tapes the window back in place over the fresh dressing
c. Removes and discards the soiled dressing and the square of plaster
d. Looks at the wound and drainage

122 A cast brace may be used to treat a fracture of the distal third of the femur. The cast brace is comprised of a thigh cuff of any type of cast material, two polycentric hinges at the knee, and a short-leg walking cast. The cast brace is an exception to the principle that is applied in the treatment of fractures by cast. The principle is that the

should include the joint above and the joint below the fracture

cast _____
_____.

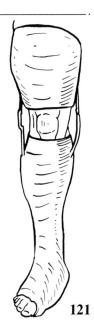

Fig. 8-20. Cast brace with thigh cuff, polycentric hinges at knee, and short-leg walking cast.

123 The cast brace is applied after the fracture fragments have been stabilized for 6 weeks in skeletal traction. The major advantages of the cast brace are that the healing period is shortened and it permits hip and knee joint motion. A cast brace is used to treat a fracture of _____

_____ .

the distal third
of the femur

124 The polycentric hinges on the cast brace must be locked when the patient is ambulatory but may be unlocked to permit flexion of the knee. The major disadvantage of a cast brace is that the patient's affected knee often swells when the patient is ambulating. The major advantages of the cast brace are:

a and b

a. It permits early ambulation
b. The patient can flex his knee
c. It eliminates the need for traction
d. It minimizes knee edema

125 The patient with a cast brace experiences minimal pain in the femur but may have difficulty with _____ .

knee edema

126 The short-leg walking cast has a walking heel, so the shoe for the patient's other foot must be built up to facilitate ambulation. When ambulating, the polycentric hinges must be (unlocked? locked?).

locked

127 The toes on the affected foot may appear somewhat darker when the patient is walking or sitting. When the patient has a cast brace, the affected foot should be observed for signs of _____

pressure sores; nerve damage; circulatory impairment

_____ , _____ ,

or _____ .

128 The patient in the next room had a spica cast put on after surgery on his right hip. The cast includes all of both legs. The bar between his legs holds the legs in a(n) _____ position The patient should be turned on the _____ leg. The patient should be observed for signs of _____

abducted

left

respiratory distress

paralytic ileus

_____ and _____ .

129 Which measures were taken to prevent pressure areas within the cast?

a, c, and d

a. Padding was applied to the bony prominences.
b. The cast was not moved until dry.
c. The nurse lifted the patient using the palms of the hands.
d. The sheet wadding was applied smoothly.

130 The nurse wonders whether the patient's plaster cast is completely dry. If it is dry, it will be _____ , _____ ,

_____ , and _____ .

131 The back of the plaster cast is not dry. To promote drying, the

nurse _____

_____ .

132 The fiberglass cast hardens or sets after being heated for several minutes under a(n) _____ .

133 The thermolabile plastic cast becomes firm as soon as it

_____ .

134 The patient in a plaster cast asks to use the bedpan. Before assisting the patient onto the bedpan, the nurse (number in order of occurrence):

_____ Turns the waterproof material back
_____ Powders the waterproof material
_____ Cuts the waterproof material to fit around the edges of the cast
_____ Slips the material under the posterior edge of the cast

135 The patient asks why the nurse is putting plastic around the edge of the cast. The nurse tells the patient that it's done to

_____

_____ .

136 The patient complains of being uncomfortable. Which of the following should the nurse report to the physician?

a. The patient feels the cast is too tight and she can't breathe (respirations are normal).
b. The patient feels too warm.
c. The patient's toes are numb.

137 The patient's daily nursing care should include:

a. Applying lotion to skin under cast
b. Applying alcohol to skin under cast
c. Checking skin for signs of rubbing
d. Washing and drying the cast

138 The patient should exercise the muscles within a cast to prevent

_____ .

139 A cast is applied by the physician to:

a. Prevent fractures
b. Prevent deformities
c. Provide rest for an inflamed joint
d. Correct a contracture

e. Immobilize the patient
f. Provide rest and support
   for bones and muscles
g. Immobilize a fracture

140 The initial assessment of the patient is important because it provides information against which the nurse can compare current observations. If the patient with a cast like the one shown in Fig. 8-19 cannot move his fingers, the nurse must know _____ _____ _____ .

whether he was able to do so before the cast was applied *(The patient may not have been able to do so for many years.)*

141 When thermolabile plastic and fiberglass materials are used, the principles of nursing care (differ greatly? remain the same?).

remain the same

142 One general principle the orthopedic surgeon generally follows when applying a cast to treat a fracture is to _____ _____ .

include the joint above and the joint below the fracture site

143 This principle is not observed when a(n) _____ is used.

cast brace

144 A cast brace is used to treat a fracture of _____ _____ and the knee (is? is not?) included in the cast.

distal third of the femur

is not

145 The major complications of a cast that the nurse should be alert for are: _____ , _____ _____ , _____ , _____ , and _____ _____ .

pressure areas; nerve damage; circulatory impairment; paralytic ileus; respiratory distress

146 Which of the following are *not* signs or symptoms of complications arising from the use of a cast?
a. Pallor   d. Pain
b. Pulselessness   e. Paresthesia
c. Paralysis

none
(All are signs or symptoms of complications.)

147 The nursing care of a patient in a plaster cast is based on:
a. Knowledge of joint motions and functions
b. Principles of body mechanics
c. Knowledge of anatomy and physiology
d. Knowledge of the individual patient's nursing care plan

All of these

148 The nursing care of a patient in a plaster cast focuses on:
a. Preparing the patient for the removal of a plaster cast
b. Observation of the patient for indications of complications
c. Prevention of complications arising from the application and use of a plaster cast
d. Helping the patient adapt to being in a plaster cast

All of these

PRINCIPLES OF NURSING CARE OF THE SURGICAL ORTHOPEDIC PATIENT

The surgical procedures utilized in the treatment of the orthopedic patient focus on restoration of function of the affected part. A surgical procedure may be done to alter the manner in which the affected part functions or to repair the part so that it functions as it did originally. Preoperatively the nursing care of the surgical patient centers on the preparation of the patient for the procedure. After surgery the appropriate nursing measures are utilized in the prevention of complications, early recognition of signs and symptoms of complications, provision of comfort measures, and assistance in the restoration of function.

CHAPTER 9

Principles of nursing care of the orthopedic patient before and after surgery

1 *Arthrodesis* is the surgical fixation of a joint that eliminates the motion of that joint. An arthrodesis is accomplished by removing the articular cartilage of the affected joint. This permits the joint surfaces to fuse together. The surgical fixation of a joint is called

arthrodesis _____ .

2 An immovable (stiff) joint is often more useful than a weak, deformed, or painful joint. By creating a stable joint, the physician restores the affected part to a more functional state. An arthrodesis results in an immovable but functional joint because the joint (can? cannot?) then be depended upon to bear weight.

can

3 If the patient has a muscular imbalance as a result of a disease such as poliomyelitis, an arthrodesis will make the joint functional and control the deformity. The physician performs an arthrodesis to _____ the position of the joint.

stabilize (fix)

4 In an arthrodesis, the joint surfaces fuse together because the _____ has been removed.

articular cartilage

5 The physician performs an arthrodesis in order to:

a, b, and d
(An immovable joint can be used to bear weight.)

a. Eliminate the motion of the joint
b. Treat a weak or painful joint
c. Prevent use of the joint
d. Treat a deformed joint

6 *Arthrotomy* is the surgical incision of a joint so that the joint may be explored. For example, the physician may explore the joint in search of a foreign body or a floating piece of torn cartilage. The main purpose of an arthrotomy is to _____ the joint.

explore

127

7 An *arthroplasty* is a surgical procedure to restore motion to a joint by creating a joint similar to the original. An arthroplasty may be done to treat a joint that has been damaged by trauma or an inflammatory disease. In an arthroplasty, joint motion is (eliminated? restored?).

restored

8 A surgical procedure to restore motion to a joint by forming a joint like the original is a(n) _____ . The surgical incision of a joint is a(n) _____ .

arthroplasty
arthrotomy

9 The physician selects an arthroplasty as the method of treatment when conservative measures have not been successful in alleviating the patient's joint pain or improving joint function. The patient's pain is the result of joint damage caused by _____ or _____ .

trauma
inflammatory disease

10 One or both of the joint surfaces may be replaced by synthetic materials in an arthroplasty. For example, in one variation of a hip arthroplasty the head of the femur is removed and a prosthesis is implanted. The joint surface is removed because it has been _____ .

damaged

11 An arthroplasty restores function as well as motion to the joint. A weight-bearing joint can again be used to bear weight since the newly constructed joint is _____ to the original joint.

similar

12 An arthrodesis _____ *joint motion;* an arthroplasty _____ *joint motion.*

eliminates
restores

13 An arthrodesis _____ *joint function;* an arthroplasty _____ _____ *joint function.*

restores or improves
restores or improves

14 An *osteotomy* is the surgical incision of a bone to correct a deformity. An osteotomy is considered to be a controlled fracture. An arthrotomy is the incision of a _____; an osteotomy is the incision of a _____ .

joint
bone

15 Osteotomy is used to correct congenital and traumatic deformities. During surgery, the physician interrupts the continuity of the bone and aligns the fragments in the corrected position. This brief description of the surgical procedure explains why an osteotomy is referred to as a(n) _____ .

controlled fracture

16 The main purpose of an osteotomy is to _____ _____ .

correct a deformity

128

17 Match the surgical procedure with the appropriate phrase:

_____ 1. Controlled fracture   a. Arthrotomy

_____ 2. Restoration of motion   b. Arthroplasty

_____ 3. Joint fusion   c. Osteotomy

_____ 4. Joint exploration   d. Arthrodesis

_____ 5. Bone incision

_____ 6. Joint incision

18 A tendon transplant is a surgical procedure that changes the attachment of a tendon. A tendon transplant may be done to change or improve function of the affected part, to replace a tendon lost by injury, and/or to correct a deformity. For example, transplanting the anterior tibial tendon to the lateral side of the dorsum of the foot may help to correct a foot deformity. A tendon transplant procedure changes the (location? attachment? function?) of the tendon.

19 A patient who has had his hand crushed in a machine is to have a tendon transplant. The nurse could reason that the transplant would:

a. Make the hand normal again

b. Help to correct the deformity

c. Replace an injured tendon

d. Improve the patient's ability to do things for himself

20 Arthrodesis, arthrotomy, arthroplasty, osteotomy, and tendon transplants are the major types of orthopedic surgical procedures. Other operative procedures are used in the treatment of fractures and soft tissue injuries and conditions. Some of these special procedures are discussed in the following chapters in relation to specific diseases and anatomical locations. When the nurse does not understand the rationale for the surgical procedure or have information regarding how it is performed, the nurse is responsible for seeking the appropriate information before caring for the patient. The following discussion presents general principles of nursing care of the surgical orthopedic patient.

21 The nursing process is generally applicable to all surgical orthopedic patients. The orthopedic nurse utilizes the nursing process as a framework to guide actions while caring for patients. The first phase of the nursing process is assessment of the patient. The *Standards of Orthopedic Nursing Practice* (p. ix) state that the nurse systematically and continuously collects data about the individual's health status. The collection of preoperative baseline data is essential, since it provides a frame of reference for postoperative comparison. The nurse assesses the patient to determine:

a. His ability to participate in activities

b. His need for immediate nursing and/or medical intervention

c. His past history of health and illness

d. His physiological status

22 The nurse assessing the orthopedic patient's current health status may use which of the following methods?

a. Interview of family members

b. Palpation of the patient's body

c. Physical examination of the patient

d. Radiographic examination

23 The physical examination of the patient is focused on the musculoskeletal system; a general physical assessment is performed to obtain baseline data regarding other body systems. The musculoskeletal examination helps to identify limitations in joint range of motion. List the terms that can be used to describe joint range of motion: _____, _____, _____, _____, _____, _____, _____, _____, and _____.

flexion; extension

hyperextension; abduction

adduction; internal rotation

external rotation; supination

pronation

24 A thorough description of any pain the patient might have will assist the physician and the nurse in determining the patient's diagnosis. (The nurse makes a *nursing* diagnosis, which is distinct from that of the physician.) List the possible characteristics of a patient's pain: _____, _____, _____, _____, _____, _____, _____, _____, _____, and _____.

location; intensity; duration; association with movement; radiation throughout body or extremity; time of onset; causative factors; usual methods of relief

25 Assessment of the neurovascular status of the extremities also provides baseline data that is useful in determining the absence, presence, or extent of neurovascular damage. The neurovascular assessment includes those aspects that were checked for indications of compartment syndrome. The ''six p's'' of compartment syndrome suggest that the patient's pain be evaluated to determine whether it is _____ or _____ and also if the pain changes with _____.

progressive; abnormal

passive motion

26 The remaining ''p's'' of compartment syndrome are _____ _____, _____, _____, and _____.

paralysis

paresthesia; pallor

pulselessness

27 An additional check of vascular status (identified in Chapter 8)

blanching test is the _____ .

28 The nurse should be able to detect gross physical deformities and to evaluate physical growth and development status. A text on pathology of the musculoskeletal system should be consulted to learn how deformities and growth and development status can be identified and described. The nurse should consider how deformities or developmental problems affect the patient's ability to participate in activities of daily living.

29 Before surgery, the nurse prepares the patient psychologically as well as physically for the surgical procedure. The psychological preparation includes exploring the patient's feelings, beliefs, expectations, and fears regarding surgery. The nurse makes observations and inferences about the patient's behavior, but the nurse must talk with the patient to validate observations and inferences. The patient's behavior may not accurately or openly reflect his reaction to the impending surgery. The nurse talks with the preoperative patient to obtain a true picture of the patient's reaction. The nurse integrates this assessment with the validation of the patient's perceptions and behavior into an identification of nursing care problems, from

nursing diagnosis which a _____ can be derived.

30 The nurse should not begin to provide information about the surgical procedure before finding out from the patient what his needs are and how they can be met. The nurse and the patient together can identify which of the patient's feelings, beliefs, problems, etc., require nursing action. The patient may have some needs that only he or members of his family can meet. The patient's nursing care

nursing action needs are emotional and physical states requiring _____

_____ .

31 The nurse and the patient can then work out together what nursing actions would be appropriate to meet his needs. For example, the nurse may find that it would be more helpful to the patient to first discuss his fears and preconceptions regarding surgical complications than to first give a logical presentation about the surgical

needs procedure. The nurse talks with the patient to identify his _____

how to meet them and _____ .

32 Number, in the order in which they occur, the steps of the nursing process as used to psychologically prepare the patient for surgery.

3 _____ The nurse validates observations and inferences with the patient.

4   _____ The nurse identifies the patient's nursing care needs.

1   _____ The nurse observes the patient's behavioral reaction to impending surgery.

5   _____ The nurse elicits from the patient what nursing actions are required to help him.

2   _____ The nurse makes inferences about the meaning of the patient's behavior.

33 Recent nursing research has shown that by using such an approach with the patient prior to surgery complications such as nausea and vomiting are reduced; that is, the psychologically prepared patient has a smoother postoperative recovery. The value of psychologically preparing the patient for surgery is that doing so tends to

postoperative complications   prevent _____ .

34 Fears of postoperative pain and changes in physical appearance are among the primary preoperative concerns of many orthopedic patients. Other orthopedic patients who have been hospitalized over an extended period of time or numerous different times because of their chronic conditions develop fears of specific aspects of treatment. For example, some patients have developed a fear of skeletal traction and are afraid they will awaken from surgery in traction. However, the nurse should not assume that every preoperative orthopedic patient has these fears. Before taking action, the nurse's inferences regarding the patient's response to the impending surgery

validated   should be _____ .

35 The patient, with the nurse's assistance, will be able to express his anxieties, beliefs, and problems, and the nurse must identify what his needs are before beginning to plan his care. The patient's

needs or problems   nursing care plan should be based on the patient's _____ .

36 The patient copes with his preoperative anxieties by employing various defense mechanisms, but with the nurse's help he will be able to identify nursing actions that could alleviate his anxieties. Nursing actions such as telling the patient about the availability of pain medications and comfort measures after surgery should be carried out only after the nurse and the patient have identified the patient's needs and the specific nursing action that would be _____

helpful or appropriate   _____ .

37 Nurses are often guilty of creating for the patient what the communication experts refer to as an information overload—we tend to provide more information than the patient can handle. The kind and amount of information to be given to the patient are established on the basis of what is needed and what would be helpful to the patient.

The appropriate information should be given in small segments. Indicate whether the following statements are true or false:

False

_____ a. The nurse should plan to tell the patient what he needs to know in one long session.

True

_____ b. The nurse should plan to talk with the patient several times to give him the needed information.

38 The physical and psychological preparation of the patient overlaps somewhat in several areas. The physical preparation of the patient includes teaching the patient how to perform activities that will be required of him postoperatively. At the same time, knowing how to do these activities may alleviate the patient's anxiety. The preoperative care and teaching principles and nursing process used for the orthopedic surgery patient may be applied in the care of the

body mechanics
(If you were unable to answer, review Section One.)

general surgery patient, just as the principles of _____ _____ are applied to all patients.

39 Preoperatively, the site of the incision must be prepared to reduce the possibility of a wound infection. The bone and tissues may become infected by bacteria entering by way of the incision in the

skin

_____ .

40 The type and extent of skin preparation depend upon the patient's condition and diagnosis, the procedure to be done, and the physician's preference. Preoperative skin preparation is done to

bone and wound infections

prevent _____ .

41 A portion of the preoperative skin preparation may be delayed until the patient is anesthetized if the patient's extremity is very painful or extremely dirty, if the patient has an open fracture, or if the extremity to be operated on is in traction. Mr. Brown has been admitted with a fractured femur. He has been placed in Russell's traction, and is scheduled for open reduction and metallic fixation

would not
(The traction cannot be removed.)

tomorrow. Mr. Brown's skin preparation (would? would not?) be completed on the nursing unit.

42 If the patient is admitted with an open fracture, he may be taken directly to the operating room, where the skin preparation is done after he is anesthetized. The preoperative skin preparation is adapted

All of these

for the patient (in traction? in severe pain? with a fracture?).

43 The condition of the patient's skin must be considered when doing the skin preparation. Those requiring special consideration are the patient with extremely dirty or greasy skin (from occupational conditions), the patient who has recently had a plaster cast removed, and the patient with a preexisting skin condition such as

133

psoriasis. Thorough cleansing of the skin could be very unpleasant and/or harmful for these patients. List the factors influencing the type and extent of the skin preparation.

a. Surgical procedures to be performed
b. Physician's preference
c. Patient's diagnosis
d. Patient's condition
e. Condition of patient's skin

a. _____

b. _____

c. _____

d. _____

e. _____

44 The area of skin prepared is determined by the surgical procedure to be performed. The operative site and the adjacent skin that might be exposed during the operation are prepared. Included in the area to be prepared are the _____

operative site

adjacent skin

_____ and _____ .

45 The first step in skin preparation is removal of all of the hair from the area. Some surgeons prefer that a depilatory be used rather than shaving the area, since it eliminates the danger of skin trauma from the razor. Shaving the area is hazardous because the skin may

traumatized (cut, nicked, or scraped)

be _____ .

46 After all the hair has been removed, the area should be scrubbed with a bacteriostatic soap solution. Some surgeons prefer that the scrub be repeated several times before the operation; others believe that once is sufficient. After the skin has been scrubbed, a sterile dressing or towel may be applied to further retard bacterial con-

cleanse the skin, prevent the growth of bacteria *(A special preparation may be necessary to remove mechanic's grease, motor oil, etc.)*

tamination. A bacteriostatic soap solution is used to (cleanse the skin? prevent the growth of bacteria? remove grease?).

47 If a foot or hand is included in the area to be prepared, the nails should be given additional attention. Any polish should be removed, and the nails should be scrubbed with a brush and trimmed.

infection

These preparatory procedures are performed to prevent _____ .

48 The plaster cast has been removed from Mrs. Smith's right leg and she is having surgery on her right knee tomorrow. Mrs. Smith's

cannot
(If you missed this, review Chapter 8.)

right leg (can? cannot?) be prepared in the usual manner.

49 Mr. Brown has sustained a very painful injury to his hand and wrist while working on his car and is to be taken from the emergency room to surgery for an open reduction. His skin preparation:

c and d

a. Can be completed in the emergency room
b. Must include cleaning his fingernails before he goes to surgery
c. Must be completed after he is anesthetized
d. Must be adapted because of the condition of his hand

50 The basic steps of the nursing process are assessment, planning, implementation, and evaluation. A brief guide to factors to be assessed has been presented and the planning of nursing care in collaboration with the patient has been discussed. The steps taken during the implementation phase—for example, skin preparation—have been presented. The impact of preoperative nursing care on the patient cannot be totally evaluated until after surgery. However, the nursing process is comprised of overlapping cycles so that postoperative planning and implementation may be initiated before the evaluation of preoperative care is completed. The nursing process framework consists of the following four basic steps: _____, _____, _____, and _____.

assess
plan; implement; evaluate

51 The nursing care of the postoperative orthopedic patient focuses on prevention of complications, early recognition of complications, providing comfort measures, assisting the patient to maintain function of the unaffected parts, and assisting the patient to regain function of the affected part. There are three types of postoperative complications for orthopedic patients; complications related to anesthesia, those related to specific orthopedic surgical procedures, and complications associated with orthopedic surgery in general. The nurse should be aware of the first type from her general surgery experiences. The complications related to specific orthopedic surgical procedures are discussed in later chapters. The following pages contain information relevant to complications generally associated with orthopedic surgery.

52 In the immediate postoperative period, the nurse must observe the patient closely for signs of hemorrhage and circulatory impairment. Many of the orthopedic surgical procedures necessitate severance or manipulation of blood vessels, both of which create the potential for hemorrhage. The primary signs of hemorrhage are changes in the patient's _____ and _____.

blood pressure
pulse

53 A large amount of sanguineous drainage is not always considered serious after orthopedic surgery although it may be indicative of hemorrhage when evaluated in isolation. The amount of bleeding should be evaluated in relation to the patient's blood pressure, pulse rate and character, and other indicators of hemorrhage. The nurse should measure the postoperative patient's _____ _____, _____, and _____ _____.

blood pressure; pulse;
amount of bleeding
(wound drainage)

54 The amount of sanguineous wound drainage should be measured at periodic intervals so that an increase in the rate of drainage can be detected before it becomes life-threatening. When the patient has had a plaster cast applied immediately after surgery, measurement of the amount of drainage is somewhat simplified. Each time the amount of drainage increases, the periphery of the drainage is outlined on the surface of the cast and marked with the time, as shown in Fig. 9-1. Mr. Smith had an arthrodesis of his left knee. On return to his room from the recovery room, his blood pressure and pulse rate are the same as they were preoperatively (132/86 and 93), and the plaster cast on his knee has an area of sanguineous drainage 4 inches in diameter over the incision. These signs (do? do not?) indicate that Mr. Smith is hemorrhaging.

do not

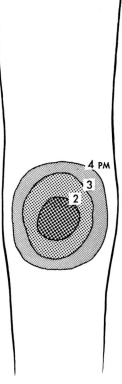

Fig. 9-1. The periphery of the drainage through the plaster cast has been outlined and marked with the appropriate hour as the drainage increased.

55 The circulation to the operated extremity must be evaluated frequently, since early recognition and treatment of circulatory impairment are essential to prevent permanent damage. The circulation to an extremity may be assessed by means of the _____ _____ .

blanching test

56 The distal portion of the operated extremity must be observed for edema if a plaster cast or constricting bandage has been applied, since it can result in permanent damage if untreated. Two nursing measures that can be instituted to prevent or reduce edema are the application of _____ and _____ _____ .

icebags; elevation of
the extremity

57 The use of icebags also has an impact on _____ .

58 Compartment syndrome is not usually seen in the postoperative orthopedic patient, since it is more frequently associated with fractures that are treated by closed reduction, casts, or traction. The complications generally associated with orthopedic surgery are

_____ , _____ , and _____ _____ .

59 Mrs. Brown has just been returned to the nursing unit following surgery. An arthrodesis was performed on her right ankle, after which a plaster cast was applied to the ankle. List the observations and measurements the nurse should make.

a. _____

b. _____

c. _____

d. _____

e. _____

60 The nurse notes that Mrs. Brown's toes are swollen, that her blood pressure and pulse rate are the same as before surgery, and that she has a large amount of drainage on her cast. The nurse recognizes that the edema must be reduced since it could lead to the development of another complication, _____

_____ . To reduce the edema and control the bleeding the

nurse should _____ _____ .

61 Nursing care measures to prevent postoperative complications such as wound infection, contractures, and pneumonia are similar to those utilized for other patients. The orthopedic patient presents a greater challenge because he is often kept in bed longer, possibly with an extremity immobilized in traction or a plaster cast. Indicate whether the following statements are true or false.

_____ a. Early recognition of complications is essential in orthopedic nursing.

_____ b. Prevention of postoperative complications is one of the important aspects of orthopedic nursing.

_____ c. Proper preoperative preparation decreases the incidence of postoperative complications.

_____ d. Prevention of a bone or wound infection is the responsibility of the physician.

62 Mr. Jones sustained a fractured right femur several years ago and has been admitted to the hospital with a diagnosis of malunion of the fracture. The surgical procedure that will be done to correct

the deformity is a(n) _____ .

63 As a part of the preoperative preparation, the nurse talks with Mr. Jones. The nurse:

a, b, and d

a. Finds out what he knows about the surgical procedure
b. Tells him what to expect after surgery
c. Explores his attitude toward current world problems
d. Tells him what will be expected of him after surgery

64 The skin at and around the incision site is prepared by

removing the hair; scrubbing the area

_____ and _____

_____ .

65 Since Mr. Jones' right foot is included in the area to be prepared,

scrubbed with a brush

trimmed

his toenails should be _____

and _____ .

prevent infection

66 These preparatory steps are taken to _____

_____ .

67 If Mr. Jones were 80 years old, a factor that would be con-

condition of his skin

sidered when preparing the operative area would be the _____

_____ .

68 During the operation, the physician inserts a bone plate and

controlled fracture

screws to immobilize the bone. An osteotomy is a _____

_____ .

69 After surgery, the nurse must observe Mr. Jones closely for indi-

hemorrhage; infection

edema; circulatory impairment

cations of _____ , _____ ,

_____ , and _____ .

70 At the time of surgery, a spica cast was applied to further im-

mobilize Mr. Jones' right leg. The physician has requested that a

To prevent foot drop.

foot board be placed on Mr. Jones' bed. Why?

71 Nursing care measures should also be taken to prevent compli-

pneumonia; decubiti;
deformities; disuse atrophy
(any two, any order)

cations such as _____ and

_____ .

72 One hour after Mr. Jones was returned to his room, the nurse

notes that the diameter of the drainage on his cast has increased by

2 inches. What other information does the nurse need to know?

His current and pre-
operative blood pressure
and pulse rate.

138

stable

stiff; immovable

73 The purpose of an arthrodesis is to create a _____, _____, or _____ joint.

arthroplasty

74 To restore motion to a joint, the surgeon may perform a(n) _____ .

osteotomy; tendon transplant

75 To correct a deformity, the surgeon may perform a(n) _____ or a(n) _____ _____ .

similar to the original joint

76 In an arthroplasty, the joint the surgeon creates is _____ _____ .

attachment of the tendon

77 In the tendon transplant procedure, the _____ _____ is changed.

a, c, d, and e

78 A tendon transplant may be performed by the surgeon to:
a. Correct a deformity
b. Change the function of the tendon
c. Replace a tendon lost by injury
d. Change the function of the affected part
e. Improve the function of the affected part

articular cartilages

fuse together

79 In an arthrodesis the _____ _____ are removed. As the wound heals, the joint surfaces _____ .

All of these

80 The nurse caring for the surgical orthopedic patient is responsible for:
a. Observing the postoperative patient for indications of complications
b. Preparing the patient preoperatively
c. Preventing complications
d. Reporting indications of complications to the physician

obtain baseline data for future comparison; identify nursing care problems or needs; make a nursing diagnosis

81 A preoperative assessment of the patient is performed in order to _____ _____ , _____ _____ , and _____ _____ .

needs or problems

pathology

82 A nursing diagnosis is different from a medical diagnosis in that the focus is on the patient's _____ rather than on _____ .

139

83 The basic steps of the nursing process are _____ ,
_____ , _____ , and _____ .

84 The nurse could evaluate the impact of the preoperative teaching
by watching to see whether postoperatively the patient _____
_____ .

85 Describe why it is important that all nursing activities be goal-
directed. Discuss your response with your instructor, classmates, or
co-workers.

Principles of nursing care of the patient having surgery on the upper extremity or shoulder

1 Motion of the upper extremity is vital for human activities of daily living. Absence, disease, or disability of any part of one or both of the upper extremities requires major adaptations in a person's activities. Consider how you would wash your face, comb your hair, or feed yourself if you had no arms or hands. This chapter is limited to considering surgical correction of conditions of the upper extremity and shoulder; other texts should be consulted for information on dealing with patients requiring major rehabilitation. Generally, active joint motion of the upper extremity (including the hand and fingers) that is smooth and painless through its complete range indicates the absence of any advanced disease or condition. As a whole,

internally

externally; toward

away from

the upper extremity can be rotated _____ or _____ and moved _____ or _____ the midline of the body.

2 Movement toward and movement away from the midline of the body are also known as _____ and

adduction

abduction

_____ .

extended

3 When your arm hangs straight at your side, it is _____ .

supination

pronation

4 The two movements unique to the forearm are _____ and _____ .

5 The wrist can be held in a neutral, flexed, or extended position; however, the two extremes of position are referred to as dorsiflexion and palmar flexion, as shown in Fig. 10-1. In dorsiflexion, the hand is moved so the back of the hand is closer to the forearm; in palmar

palm

flexion the _____ of the hand is moved closer to the forearm.

141

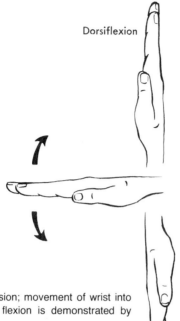

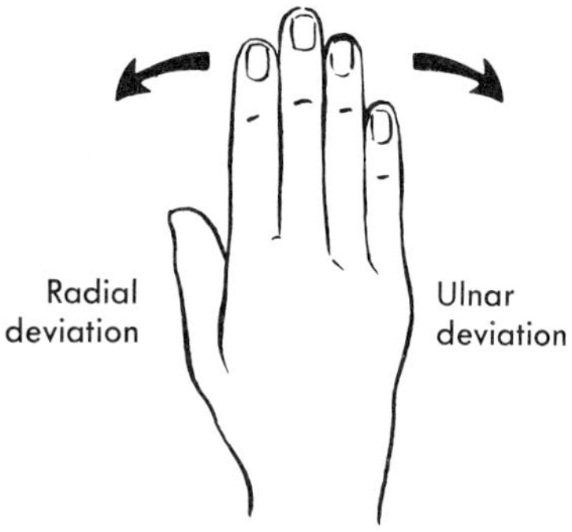

Dorsiflexion

Radial deviation

Ulnar deviation

Fig. 10-2. Radial and ulnar deviation at wrist. Wrist is examined for this movement with forearm pronated.

Fig. 10-1. Wrist in extension; movement of wrist into dorsiflexion and palmar flexion is demonstrated by arrows.

Palmar flexion

6 The position of the hand in relation to the forearm should also be examined for radial and ulnar deviation, as shown in Fig. 10-2. In radial deviation the hand is moved toward the side of the forearm where the _____ is located. In ulnar deviation, the hand is moved toward the side of the forearm where the _____ is located.

radius
ulna

7 On assessment, the nurse should observe the patient's wrist and forearm movements to assure that the following motions are possible: _____ and _____, _____ and _____ deviation, _____ and _____ flexion.

supination; pronation
radial; ulnar; dorsiflexion
plantar

8 Each of the fingers can be flexed or extended as a whole or at either the proximal or distal interphalangeal joints. Deformities such as are seen in the arthritic hand may be manifested by flexion contractures at the distal interphalangeal joints. Deformity may also be present in the metacarpophalangeal joints. If contracture deformities of the fingers are inevitable, it is best that they occur with the fingers in (extension? flexion?).

flexion

9 The nursing care of a patient with diseased, deformed, or injured hand or fingers focuses on the preservation and restoration of function. The ability to use the hand is vital for the activities of daily living, as well as the source of income for many patients. The basic function of the hand is the ability to _____

pinch or grasp
(If you were unable to answer, review Chapter 2.)

_____ .

10 Fingers and hands are often injured in accidents both at home and at work. The extent of injury varies in these accidents. A simple laceration may have been incurred, a tendon may have been severed, or the entire hand may have been badly mangled in a machine. The medical and nursing care of these patients is directed toward

preservation; restoration

_____ and _____

of function.

11 Reconstructive surgery on the hand may be done immediately after the injury or at a later date. One of the surgical procedures used to correct a deformity or improve function is a _____

tendon transplant
(If you were unable to answer, review Chapter 9.)

_____ .

12 In addition to hand injuries, deformities may result from diseases such as arthritis. Although it may not be possible to correct these deformities, surgery may be performed to improve the

function

_____ of the hand.

13 Surgery may also be done on the hand or fingers to remove growths or tumors. Other indications for hand surgery are to

correct deformities;
improve function

_____ and to _____

_____ .

14 Regardless of the type of procedure to be performed, meticulous preoperative skin preparation of the hand and fingers is done to prevent loss of function resulting from wound infection. The preoperative skin preparation is adapted accordingly but should include:

a, b, and c
(Skin preparation may be done after the patient is anesthetized in surgery.)

a. Trimming the fingernails
b. Removing grease or dirt
c. Removing any rings
d. Washing with iodine solution

15 Dupuytren's contracture is a flexion deformity of one or more fingers of the involved hand. The contracture results from chronic inflammation of the palmar fascia with progressive fibrosis. The deformity resulting from Dupuytren's contracture is corrected by excising the abnormal palmar fascia. Dupuytren's contracture is

chronic inflammation
of the palmar fascia

caused by _____

_____ .

16 Two inflammatory conditions that result in finger deformities are

143

Dupuytren's contracture
arthritis

_____

and _____ .

17 One of the more common growths of the hand is a *ganglion*, a benign cystic structure connected to a joint capsule. Like Dupuytren's contracture, a ganglion is treated by surgical _____ .

excision

18 Dupuytren's contracture involves the _____ .
A ganglion is connected to a _____ .

palmar fascia
joint capsule

19 The postoperative nursing care is modified for the individual patient and depends upon the type and extent of the surgical procedure and the patient's unique needs. In the previous chapter it was pointed out that the major objectives of the postoperative nursing care of orthopedic patients are:

a. Prevention of complications

b. Early recognition of complications

c. Provision of comfort measures

d. Assisting the patient to maintain function of the unaffected part

e. Assisting the patient to regain function of the affected part

a. _____
_____

b. _____
_____

c. _____
_____

d. _____
_____

e. _____
_____

20 Postoperatively, the nurse must check the operated fingers and hand frequently to see if the circulation is adequate. Impaired circulation must be recognized and treated promptly to prevent permanent damage. The adequacy of the circulation to the operated hand is evaluated by:

All of these
(Note: All of these apply to the hand or fingers on which the surgery was performed.)

a. Checking the skin color
b. Asking the patient to move his fingers
c. Doing the blanching test
d. Taking the patient's pulse

21 The surgical dressing used on the hand or fingers depends upon the type of surgery performed. A plaster cast may be utilized to immobilize the wrist joint and/or to maintain a functional position of the fingers, hand, or wrist. Indicate which statements are true and which are false.

False

True

True

_____ a. There is no treatment for circulatory impairment.
_____ b. Prolonged circulatory impairment can result in permanent damage.
_____ c. The nurse is responsible for recognizing signs of circulatory impairment.

144

22 A plaster cast may be applied after hand or finger surgery:

a and b

a. To keep the patient from moving his wrist
b. To hold the hand and fingers in the proper position for healing
c. To prevent swelling of the fingers
d. To keep the patient from touching the wound

23 Edema can develop within a plaster cast and cause circulatory impairment. The possibility of edema developing and causing circulatory impairment is increased if immediately after surgery a

plaster cast; constrictive
bandage

_____ or _____ _____ has been applied.

24 Rather than waiting for edema to develop, the nurse should prevent it by elevating the patient's hand. Any means may be used to elevate the hand, but the hand must be held higher than the heart to be effective.

25 The patient's hand can be elevated on pillows, placed in a sling, or suspended and supported in an upright position as shown in Fig. 10-3. To prevent edema, the hand must be held _____

higher than the heart

_____ .

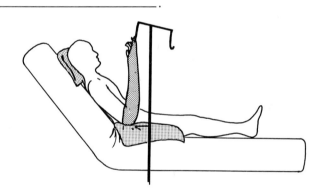

Fig. 10-3. The patient's arm is suspended from an intravenous standard to elevate the hand.

26 If, while checking the circulation to the patient's hand, the nurse notes that the fingers and/or hand are becoming edematous, an ice-bag should be used to reduce the swelling. Indications of impaired circulation are:

a. Cool or cold skin
b. Pale or cyanotic skin color
c. Inability to move previously movable fingers
d. Sluggish return of blood in blanching test
e. Patient complaints of numbness or pain
(any four, any order)

a. _____
_____

b. _____
_____

c. _____
_____

d. _____
_____

145

27 Edema of the hand and fingers can be prevented by:

a, c, and d
*(c and d are applications of
the principles of care of the
patient in a plaster cast.)*

a. Elevating the operated hand on pillows

b. Loosening the dressing

c. Applying an icebag

d. Encouraging the patient to move his fingers

28 The nurse should review the physician's orders for limitations of movement. If there are no limitations, the patient should be encouraged to move the fingers frequently to prevent joint stiffness (and loss of function). While the hand is at rest, it should be held in a functional position. The patient is instructed to move his fingers frequently because doing so will prevent _____

joint stiffness

edema

_____ and _____ .

29 After the sutures are removed, the physician often requests physical therapy treatments or active exercises for the patient. The treatments and exercises will assist the patient in regaining function of the affected fingers or hand. A functional position of the hand and fingers would be one in which:

c

a. The fingers are extended and the thumb flexed

b. The fingers are flexed and the thumb extended

c. The thumb and fingers are partially flexed and opposed

30 Surgical procedures are performed upon the wrist to correct a deformity, to restore motion and strength, to stabilize the joint, or to remove a growth. The functional position of the wrist is extension. If fusion of the wrist is necessary to maintain correction of the deformity, the physician will place the wrist in the functional position. The surgical procedure that eliminates the motion of a joint

arthrodesis

is a(n) _____ . If the patient has a progressive disease that will result in fusion of the joints, the nurse should sup-

extension

port the wrist in the functional position, which is _____ .

31 Total wrist arthroplasty is now being performed on a limited basis, to restore pain-free, stable motion at the wrist. Total wrist arthroplasty is indicated in patients with significant disability such as loss of strength and/or motion due to rheumatoid or post-traumatic arthritis. Total wrist arthroplasty is performed to restore joint

motion; strength

_____ and _____ .

32 A total wrist arthroplasty, although relatively untested, is preferable for many patients to wrist arthrodesis. Wrist arthrodesis may

motion

be effective in restoring partial function but wrist _____ is lost.

rheumatoid or
post-traumatic arthritis

33 Wrist deformity or disability is often caused by _____

_____ .

34 The surgical procedure is intricate because of the caution that must be taken to preserve blood vessels and nerves that supply the hand and fingers. After the surgery is completed, the surgeon usually applies a bulky dressing to the forearm and wrist. The dressing may incorporate a splint to prevent wrist motion until primary healing has occurred. This description implies that the nurse should check postoperatively the total wrist replacement patient for signs of

circulatory impairment; nerve damage

_____ or _____
_____ .

35 The major reasons for performing a total wrist arthroplasty are:

a and b

a. To correct deformity caused by arthritis
b. To restore joint function
c. To improve appearance of wrist
d. To repair fractured bones

36 Although the symptoms of carpal tunnel syndrome are paresthesia and pain in the hand, the cause originates in the wrist. Carpal tunnel syndrome is caused by compression of the median nerve by swollen tendon sheaths under the carpal ligament. Surgical decompression usually results in complete return of function of the nerve and the affected fingers. Carpal tunnel syndrome is caused by:

b and c

a. An edematous median nerve
b. Compression of the median nerve
c. Edematous tendon sheaths

surgical decompression

37 Carpal tunnel syndrome is treated by _____
_____ .

38 The surgical dressing applied to the wrist depends upon the type of surgery that was performed. The dressing may be heavy enough to immobilize the wrist, or it may include a splint to immobilize and support the wrist. If prolonged immobilization is anticipated, a plaster cast may be applied to the wrist. The purposes of a wrist splint

immobilize; support

are to _____ and _____ the joint.

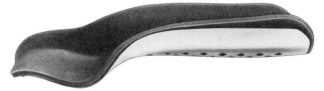

Fig. 10-4. A foam-padded forearm splint used to immobilize and support the wrist. (Courtesy Zimmer • USA, Warsaw, Ind.)

39 After wrist surgery, the nurse must check the patient's fingers for indications of circulatory impairment. The impairment could be caused by injury to a blood vessel at the time of surgery or by

147

pressure from a heavy dressing, splint, or plaster cast. The nurse should check the fingers on the operative hand for skin _____ and _____ and loss of _____ and/or _____ .

40 Which part of Fig. 10-5 demonstrates the proper way to support and elevate the hand or wrist postoperatively? _____

Fig. 10-5

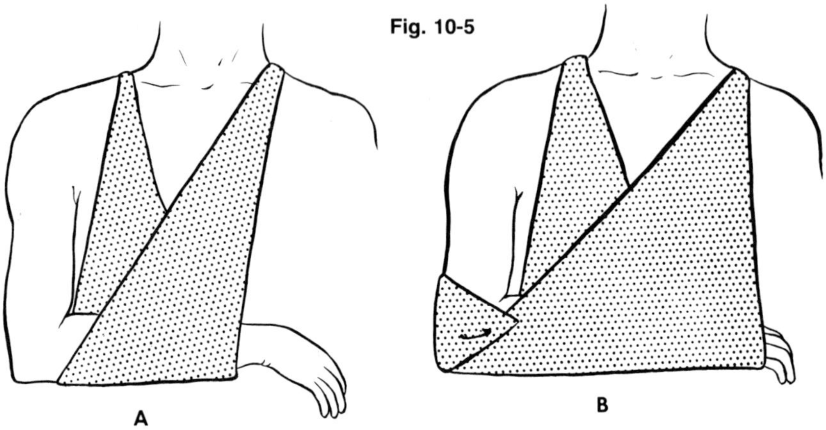

A   B

41 Total elbow arthroplasty is being done on a limited basis to restore motion to the elbow joint. Trauma and arthritis are two conditions that can lead to destruction of the joint surfaces with accompanying loss of pain-free motion. The term total elbow arthroplasty implies that the surgical procedure _____ .

42 Extension and flexion of the elbow joint can be restored after trauma or disease by means of _____ _____ .

43 The postoperative complications of total elbow arthroplasty are similar to those of other total joint replacement procedures. Possible postoperative complications include _____ _____ , _____ , _____ _____ , _____ _____ , and _____ .

44 Surgery is performed on the shoulder to repair the joint after injury, to correct a deformity, or to remove a growth. Athletes and young people frequently injure their shoulders in physical activities, with the most common result being a dislocated shoulder. The repeatedly dislocated shoulder eventually requires surgery. Indications for shoulder surgery include (congenital deformities? traumatic dislocations? inflammatory disorders? tumors?).

45 To treat recurrent dislocations, the Putti-Platt procedure is one of the numerous procedures that can be utilized to stabilize the shoulder and to prevent future dislocations by limiting external rotation. The Putti-Platt procedure:

b, d, and e

a. Is used to correct deformities
b. Prevents further dislocations
c. Is used to remove growths
d. Limits external rotation
e. Stabilizes the shoulder joint

46 An adducted arm position must be maintained for approximately 3 weeks after the Putti-Platt procedure to permit healing. The arm is adducted with the elbow flexed and is strapped to the patient's body. After the strapping is removed, the physician usually prescribes a program of active exercises to assist the patient in regaining motion and strengthening the shoulder. The affected arm is immobilized postoperatively:

c

a. To prevent infection
b. To prevent external rotation
c. To allow the joint structures to heal

47 Postoperatively, a plaster cast is occasionally used to immobilize the arm in abduction. After the Putti-Platt procedure, the arm of the affected side is strapped to the patient's body in _____.

adduction

A plaster cast may be used after other procedures to hold the arm in

abduction

_____.

48 After shoulder surgery, the arm is always immobilized:

c

a. In adduction
b. In abduction
c. In the position prescribed
d. In external rotation

49 The nursing care of the patient who has had shoulder surgery is similar to that of the patient who has had hand surgery. The patient's hand and fingers must be observed for signs of _____

circulatory impairment

_____.

50 Although the blood supply may be stopped at the shoulder, circulation to the fingers can be readily evaluated by means of the

blanching test

_____.

51 Surgical excision is the usual method of treatment of:

b and d

a. Carpal tunnel syndrome

149

b. Dupuytren's contracture
c. Putti-Platt disease
d. Ganglionic cyst

52 The patient has had surgery on his left wrist; the nurse is observing him closely for indications of circulatory impairment. Which of these observations are indications of possible impairment?

a. Patient can move all of his fingers freely.
b. Patient complains of numbness in his left fingers.
c. Patient's right radial pulse is 80.
d. Patient's right fingers are cool to touch.
e. Patient's left radial pulse is weak.

53 After hand, wrist, or finger surgery, the complication of edema

is

(is? is not?) preventable.

54 Complete the table by writing in the functional position of the part named:

a. Extension
b. Slight flexion
c. Slight abduction

a. Wrist— _____
b. Fingers— _____
c. Arm— _____

pinch or grasp

55 The most vital function of the hand is the ability to _____
_____ .

56 The reasons for performing orthopedic surgery on the upper extremity are to:

a. Improve function (stabilize joint)
b. Correct deformity
c. Repair joint injury
d. Remove growth

a. _____
b. _____
c. _____
d. _____

57 Movement of the fingers following hand or wrist surgery should be encouraged, unless restricted by the physician, in order to pre-

joint stiffness; edema

vent _____ and _____ .

58 Postoperative edema of the fingers and hand can also be pre-

elevating the hand

vented by _____ .

59 When the hand or wrist is elevated or immobilized, it should

supported in a
functional position

be _____
_____ .

60 The nursing care of the patient having surgery on the upper

preservation of function;
restoration of function

extremity must be centered on the _____
_____ and the _____
_____ .

150

Principles of nursing care of the patient having surgery on the lower extremity or hip joint

1 The nursing and medical care of the patient having surgery on the lower extremity or hip is centered on assisting the patient to function normally. Weight-bearing and ambulation are the main functions of the lower extremity and hip joint. The lower extremities and hip joints are used primarily to _____ and to _____ .

walk; stand

2 Surgical procedures are performed on the lower extremity and hip joint to permit the patient to ambulate and to bear weight comfortably and correctly. When the patient's lower extremities or hip joints are unstable or painful because of congenital deformities, disease, or injury, the patient develops protective posture and movement patterns that are deleterious. A limp resulting from painful feet, for example, places additional stress on the hip joints that can lead to joint damage. Surgical intervention enables the patient to ambulate and bear weight _____ and _____ .

comfortably
correctly

3 Surgery of the foot may be indicated to remove growths such as tumors and abnormal bony overgrowths, to repair the damage caused by disease or injury, or to correct deformities resulting from congenital defects, disease, or injury. The overall goal of surgical treatment of the foot is to _____ _____ _____ .

permit the patient to ambulate
and bear weight com-
fortably and correctly

4 The principles of pre- and postoperative nursing care are adapted as needed when the patient has surgery on the foot. The preoperative skin preparation of the foot is essentially the same as that for the hand. The steps of the preoperative skin preparation of the foot should consist of:

b, c, and d

a. Soaking in an antiseptic solution
b. Removal of all of the hair

151

c. Cleaning and trimming the nails

d. Scrubbing with a brush

5 After surgery, the toes of the operated foot must be checked frequently by the nurse for signs of circulatory impairment, just as the fingers are checked after hand surgery. Indicate which points the nurse should check.

a, b, and d

a. Response of the nails to the blanching test

b. Patient's ability to move his toes

c. Dryness of the skin

d. Skin color and temperature

6 A *bunionectomy* is a surgical procedure to remove an exostosis, a bony overgrowth, that has made weight-bearing and walking uncomfortable for the patient. Surgical procedures may be done on the foot:

a, b, c, and d

a. To correct deformities

b. To remove growths

c. To restore functioning after a disease

d. To restore functioning after an injury

e. To supplement functioning by the addition of digits

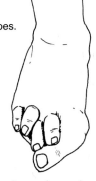

Fig. 11-1. The patient's foot is deformed by a bunion and hammer toes.

7 Because of the deformities caused by bunions, the patient who requires a bunionectomy may also require corrective surgery on the toes. If so, both procedures are done at the same time. Bunions are

bony overgrowths

_____ .

8 A bunionectomy is performed to:

a. Remove bony overgrowth

b. Correct deformities

a. _____

b. _____

9 After surgery the patient remains in bed with his feet elevated to prevent edema. Several days after surgery, the physician may permit the bunionectomy patient to get out of bed. Immediately after sur-

is not
edema

gery, the bunionectomy patient (is? is not?) permitted to ambulate in order to prevent _____ .

10 After surgery the patient's toes are very sensitive and uncomfortable, and nursing measures must be taken to protect them. A bed cradle or other device placed on the patient's bed will keep the covers from coming into contact with the patient's toes and will facilitate observation of the toes. The aims of nursing care are:

a, b, and d

a. To prevent edema
b. To protect the toes from being traumatized
c. To observe the toes for signs of hemorrhage
d. To observe the patient for signs of complications

11 The bunionectomy patient should be taught to walk with a walker as soon as the physician has prescribed walking with partial or no weight-bearing on the operated foot. List the nursing actions, other than observations, utilized in the postoperative care of the bunionectomy patient.

a. Elevate feet
b. Protect feet with bed cradle
c. Teach patient to use walker

a. _____

b. _____

c. _____

12 Indicate which statements are true and which are false.

False

_____ a. The bunionectomy patient is permitted to ambulate the day of surgery.

False

_____ b. All bunionectomy patients should be taught to use corrective shoes.

True (*Edema is a complication.*)

_____ c. The bunionectomy patient's feet are elevated to prevent complications.

True

_____ d. The bunionectomy patient usually has deformed toes along with bunions.

13 Match the surgical procedure with the appropriate phrase.

c
a
b

_____ 1. Arthrodesis   a. Creation of a joint
_____ 2. Arthroplasty   b. Exploration of a joint
_____ 3. Arthrotomy   c. Fusion of a joint

14 Congenital defects, diseases, and/or injuries can weaken the ankle and make it undependable and painful for weight-bearing and walking. The ankle can be made more stable by the appropriate surgical procedure. For example, fusion of the ankle by arthrodesis is one approach to stabilizing the ankle. An unstable or painful ankle

congenital defect

disease; injury

may result from _____ ,

_____ , or _____ .

15 A plaster cast that extends from the patient's toes to above the knee is applied after an ankle arthrodesis is performed. The nursing care of the ankle arthrodesis patient utilizes the principles of care of a patient in a plaster cast, with particular attention given to the amount of surgical wound drainage on the cast. When checking the amount of drainage, the nurse must:

a and c

a. Mark the edges of the drainage at periodic intervals so that the amount can be calculated
b. Remember that there should not be very much drainage
c. Evaluate the amount in relation to the patient's blood pressure and pulse rate and character

16 The nurse should observe the arthrodesis patient for signs of

hemorrhage; circulatory impairment

_____ and _____ _____ .

17 In the immediate postoperative period, swelling should be controlled by placing icebags next to the cast. The nursing care of the arthrodesis patient focuses on the _____

early recognition

prevention

_____ and _____ of complications.

18 The arthrodesis patient is not usually allowed to bear weight on the operated ankle for at least 6 weeks, although he may be allowed to walk with a walker or crutches. The physician may change the patient's cast 6 weeks after surgery and put a walking heel on the new cast so that the patient can bear weight when he walks. Within the limitations specified by the physician for the individual patient, the arthrodesis patient:

b and d

a. Can ambulate as desired
b. Can ambulate with crutches or a walker
c. Can bear weight on the newly operated ankle
d. Can sit in a chair with his ankle elevated

19 An unstable ankle may result from:

All of these

a. Injury to the ankle
b. A congenital defect
c. Malunion of a fracture
d. Disease of the ankle bones

20 Surgical procedures on the foot and ankle enable the patient to function normally, often for the first time, so that the patient is able

walk (ambulate); bear weight

able to _____ and _____ .

21 The hinge joint structure of the knee predisposes it to injury since the joint permits only a small amount of rotation and lateral motion when the knee is flexed. The muscles and ligaments must be strong to bind the joint components together. Attempts to rotate the

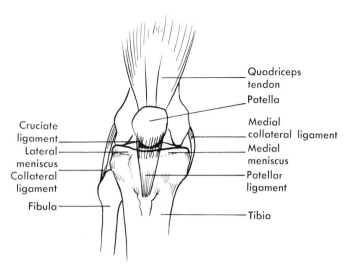

Fig. 11-2. Basic anatomic structure of knee. Note that collateral ligaments prevent the femoral condyles from moving laterally across tibial plateau.

injury to the knee

extended leg can result in _____

_____ .

22 The *menisci* (semilunar cartilages) are structures of the knee that are often traumatized. *Meniscectomy*—removal of one or both of the menisci—may be performed if the knee is repeatedly injured. Bunionectomy is the removal of _____ .

bony overgrowths

menisci (semilunar cartilages)

Menisectomy is the removal of the _____

_____ .

23 Injuries to the menisci are typically sustained by forced internal rotation of the femur on the tibia while the knee is flexed and the foot is firmly placed on the ground. One indication for knee surgery is

injury

_____ to the menisci.

24 Since other pathology may be responsible for loss of knee joint function, diagnosis may be facilitated by an *arthrogram* or an *arthroscopic examination* of the knee joint. An arthrogram utilizes air and contrast media to aid visualization of the structures of the knee on x-ray. An arthroscope can be utilized to directly visualize the knee synovia, menisci, cruciate ligaments, articular cartilage, and the undersurface of the patella.

25 These diagnostic procedures may reveal that one or more of the knee structures has been injured. Such an injury may require surgical repair. To diagnose joint injury or damage, the physician may per-

arthrogram

form a(n) _____ and/or explore the joint

arthroscope

with a(n) _____ .

155

26 Degenerative joint diseases such as osteoarthritis and rheumatoid arthritis (discussed in a later chapter) often damage the joint structures and lead to painful weight bearing and loss of motion. Indications for surgery on the knee include _____ and

_____ .

injury

degenerative joint disease

27 Degenerative joint disease may involve one or both of the femoral condyles, and/or the tibial surface, and at times the patella. Severe damage of the joint surfaces from degenerative joint disease is one indication for a total joint replacement of the knee. Total knee joint replacement may be performed to reduce pain, improve range of motion, improve joint stability and function, or correct joint deformity. If the total knee replacement is bicondylar, (one? both?) femoral condyles are replaced.

both

28 The objectives for total knee joint replacement include:
a. Correction of varus instability
b. Improvement in range of motion
c. Change in patient's gait
d. Relief of pain
e. Repair of injured ligaments

a, b, c, and d
(Correction of gait may be necessary to prevent injury to hip joint.)

29 Before the patient has knee surgery, the nurse should teach him how to do quadriceps-setting, isometric contraction, and leg-raising exercises. It is helpful if the patient learns how to perform these exercises during the preoperative period since he will be required to do them after surgery to strengthen the knee. Before surgery, the patient practices doing _____

_____ , _____ ,

and _____ exercises.

quadriceps-setting

isometric contraction

leg-raising

30 The preoperative nursing care of the patient having knee surgery should include:

a. _____
_____

b. _____
_____

c. _____
_____

a. Teaching the patient how to do exercises
b. Psychological preparation of the patient
c. Skin preparation of the operative area

31 The preoperative preparation of the patient for total knee replacement includes the collection of preoperative baseline data such as x-rays of the involved knee, electrocardiogram, chest x-ray, and blood chemistry and cell studies. These data must be available so the patient's preoperative status and postoperative progress can be accurately evaluated. The four basic elements of preoperative prepara-

skin preparation; data
collection; psychological
preparation; patient
teaching

tion of the total knee replacement patient are: _____
_____ , _____ ,
_____ ,
and _____ .

32 Wound infection of the total knee replacement is extremely serious because it may require extended antibiotic therapy, surgery to debride the wound, or removal of the replacement components, leaving the patient with an unstable or nonfunctional knee joint. Many surgeons prescribe large doses of antibiotics to be given just before the patient is taken to the operating room to assist in the prevention of infection. The nurse may also be responsible for making certain that the appropriate antibiotic wound irrigating solution is available for use during the surgical procedure. Postoperative wound infection is prevented by _____
_____ and _____
_____
_____ .

giving antibiotics preoperatively; irrigating the wound
with antibiotic solution
during surgery

33 There is a wide variety of knee components available for use in the total knee replacement procedure. The physician will request variations in nursing care according to which components are used. The components used in the total knee replacement procedure are cemented into place with surgical bone cement (methylmethacrylate). At the time the components are cemented into place the patient may react physiologically. A transient drop in blood pressure and a change in pulse rate may be noted. Usually these physiological changes are only temporary and are self-correcting.

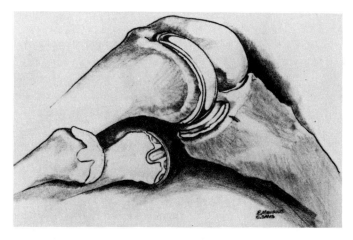

Fig. 11-3. Unicondylar replacement of femoral and tibial articular surfaces of knee joint in total joint replacement. Lower left portion of drawing demonstrates how femoral component fits into femoral condyle. (Courtesy Richards Mfg. Co., Memphis.)

34 The surgical dressing placed on the knee after surgery is a cast or pressure dressing to retard oozing and bleeding into the joint and swelling. A pressure dressing, a posterior splint, or other means of support is also used to prevent flexion or motion of the knee. The purposes of the pressure dressing are _____ _____ , _____ , _____ _____ .

to retard oozing and bleeding into the joint; to prevent edema; to prevent flexion or motion of the knee

35 Edema of the operative knee can also be prevented by _____ _____ or _____ _____ .

elevating the leg; applying icebags

36 During the immediate postoperative period, the operated leg must be held in extension at all times. Elevation of the operated knee must be done carefully to assure that the desired position is maintained. The operated knee must be held in (flexion? extension?).

extension

37 The patient should be observed postoperatively for signs of circulatory impairment and damage to the peroneal nerve. Damage to the peroneal nerve is manifested by decreased sensation over the dorsum of the foot. The possible postoperative complications of knee surgery include _____ _____ , _____ , _____ _____ , and _____ _____ .

bleeding into the joint; edema; circulatory impairment; peroneal nerve damage

38 Signs of circulatory impairment and peroneal nerve damage should be reported promptly because they can cause _____ _____ .

permanent damage

39 Since total knee replacement is a much more extensive procedure than meniscectomy, the patient is open to several additional possible complications. Early in the postoperative phase the patient may develop a hematoma, skin necrosis, or superficial infection of the wound. Indicate which statements are true.

a, b, and d

a. The meniscectomy patient may develop a wound infection.
b. The total knee replacement patient may develop wound site skin necrosis.
c. Circulatory impairment postoperatively is not a potential complication of knee surgery.
d. Total knee replacement infection may result in loss of joint motion.

40 Postoperative thrombophlebitis of the affected extremity poses a serious threat to the total knee replacement patient. The physician may prescribe anticoagulant therapy as a preventive measure. When the patient is on anticoagulant therapy, his prothrombin time must be monitored closely. Knowledge of anticoagulant therapy leads the nurse to also monitor the patient for indication of postoperative

hemorrhage _____ .

41 Postoperative hemorrhage is a very real possibility because the bone is penetrated when the sites are prepared for the placement of the components; the anticoagulant therapy contributes to the hazard by removing the natural physiological protection. The possible immediate postoperative complications of total knee replacement include: _____ , _____ ,

hemorrhage; thrombophlebitis; circulatory impairment; peroneal nerve damage; skin necrosis; hematoma formation; superficial wound infection

_____ , _____

_____ , _____ ,

_____ , and _____

_____

_____ .

42 At the time the wound is closed, the surgeon may insert a drain in the wound, which is connected to mild suction for the first 24 to 48 hours after surgery. The amount of drainage as well as the patient's

hemorrhage vital signs should be monitored for indications of _____ .

43 Control of wound edema and hemorrhage can be assisted by the

icebags or pressure dressing application of _____

_____ .

44 The patient begins doing quadriceps-setting, isometric, and leg-raising exercises immediately after surgery since he may not be permitted out of bed until the muscles have regained the strength necessary to maintain extension. Dorsiflexion of the ankle should also be encouraged. When the physician directs, the patient is allowed to ambulate with crutches, but he is not permitted to bear weight on the operated knee. Exercises are done postoperatively in order to

strengthen the muscles _____ .

45 The physician adjusts the patient's weight-bearing limitations and knee motion as the wound heals and the muscles are strengthened. The patient gradually progresses from non–weight-bearing to partial and then full weight-bearing on the affected extremity. The progression of weight-bearing depends upon the surgical procedure performed. Until the physician directs otherwise, the operated leg

extended must be maintained in the _____ position.

46 During the intermediate recovery phase the total knee replacement patient begins flexion of the affected knee joint during ambulation and while sitting. Flexion contractures may develop if the patient is permitted to place a pillow under his knee when he is in bed. Abrupt flexion of the knee may result in joint subluxation. Delayed healing may also become apparent during this phase. Intermediate postoperative complications include _____

_____ , _____ ,

and _____ .

47 One of the most serious complications of total knee replacement surgery is infection around the replacement components. Such an infection may not develop until the late postoperative phase. Infection around the replacement components can be serious because:

a. The patient may lose the function of the joint
b. The prosthetic components must always be removed
c. The patient will require an arthrodesis of the knee after the infection is treated
d. The patient may go into septic shock

48 During the late postoperative phase loosening of one or more of the replacement components can occur. This is critical for the patient because the only treatment available at this time is surgical removal of the loose component. An arthrodesis may then be performed. This permits weight-bearing; however, the affected leg may be shorter and the knee's motion is lost. Two critical complications that may occur late in the recovery phase of total knee replacement are

_____

_____ and _____

_____ .

49 Some patients experience malalignment of the knee components, which results in a valgus deformity. This may be seen with a recurring displacement of the patella. At other times, total dislocation of the components may occur because of severe joint instability or improper seating of the joint replacement components. These complications require corrective surgery to permit _____

_____ or _____ .

50 Like the other late complications, fatigue fracture at the medial tibial cortex occurs infrequently. However, the nurse must constantly be alert for indications of complications. Reportable signs of late phase complications would include: _____ , _____

_____ , _____ ,

_____ , _____

_____ , and _____ .

51 Antibiotic therapy is continued after surgery as a precautionary measure. Dressing changes should be performed with meticulous aseptic technique to prevent wound contamination. For what other possible complication is a medication prescribed? _____

52 The late phase postoperative complications that may occur include _____

_____ , _____

_____ , _____

_____ ,

_____ , and _____

_____ .

53 The nursing care of the total knee replacement patient is very
much like that of patients who have had other surgical procedures
performed. The patient may sit up or turn from side to side as desired except during the immediate postoperative phase, when the
affected limb must be elevated to prevent the development of

_____ .

54 The total knee replacement patient may receive parenteral fluids
until the possibility of hemorrhagic shock has passed, until the patient is able to take ample amounts of oral fluids, and/or to permit
intravenous administration of antibiotics. If the patient's blood pressure decreases, his pulse rate increases, and his hematocrit and
hemoglobin values are low the evening of surgery, the surgeon may

wish to intravenously administer _____

_____ .

55 Indicate which statements about the nursing care of the patient
having surgery of the lower extremity are true and which are false.

_____ a. One aim of nursing care is to observe the patient for
indications of a skin reaction.

_____ b. One goal of nursing care is to control edema.

_____ c. One goal of nursing care is to assist the patient to resume weight-bearing and walking as the physician
directs.

_____ d. One aim of nursing care is to observe the patient for
indications of complications.

_____ e. One aim of nursing care is to keep the patient completely immobile.

56 The hip joint is continuously submitted to the stresses of weight-
bearing and walking and, therefore, is prone to injury and disease.
Arthroplasty, arthrodesis, and osteotomy are the surgical procedures
performed to stabilize the hip joint and relieve the patient's pain.
Match the surgical procedure with the appropriate phrase.

_____ 1. Osteotomy   a. Fusion of a joint

_____ 2. Arthroplasty   b. A controlled fracture

_____ 3. Arthrodesis   c. Creation of a new joint

57 The most prevalent diseases of the hip joint are degenerative joint diseases and inflammatory diseases, both of which are more common in the elderly. Injuries to the hip joint, especially fractures, are also associated with advanced age. The reasons for hip surgery are _____ or _____ .

disease; injury

58 Femoral fractures are typically treated surgically when the fracture involves the head, neck, or intertrochanteric region. The surgical treatment can be open reduction with metallic fixation or arthroplasty with insertion of a prosthesis. The surgical procedures that can be performed on the hip are _____ , _____ , _____ , and _____ .

arthroplasty
arthrodesis; osteotomy
open reduction

59 There are numerous principles of nursing care that are applicable when caring for the hip surgery patient regardless of the surgical procedure performed. Nursing care is adapted for the individual patient within a framework of the principles, the constraints imposed by the specific procedure, the physician's directions, and the patient's unique needs. Nursing care of the hip surgery patient is focused on the prevention of complications related to the surgical procedure, to the administration of anesthesia, and to immobilization, assisting the patient to maintain function of the unaffected extremities, and assisting the patient to regain function of the affected extremity. The factors influencing the nursing care of the hip surgery patient are _____ _____ , _____ , _____ , and _____ .

nursing care principles; the specific procedure; physician's directions; patient's needs

60 The possible complications of hip surgery attributable to the administration of anesthesia and immobilization tend to overlap. For example, postoperative hypostatic pneumonia is associated with both the anesthesia and inactivity. The nursing care utilized in the prevention of these complications incorporates the principles governing the prevention of complications related to the surgical procedure and body mechanics. Nursing care of the hip surgery patient is guided by an integrated set of principles and is centered on prevention of complications associated with _____ , _____ , and _____ .

anesthesia
immobilization; the surgical procedure

61 Most arthroplasty procedures except total hip joint replacement necessitate prolonged periods of bed rest with immobilization of the operative hip joint to prevent dislocation or subluxation of the hip joint. Indicate whether the following statements are true or false.

162

_____ a. Dislocation is movement of a bone out of its normal joint position.

_____ b. Subluxation is movement of a bone into position behind a joint.

62 The subluxation of a joint is a partial or incomplete dislocation. If the head of the femur is dislocated, it is moved (into? out of?) the acetabulum.

63 Postoperatively, the physician will specify the degree of abduction and type of rotation appropriate for the patient. Abduction splints, plaster casts, and/or traction are often used to maintain the degree of abduction. Abduction is movement (away from? toward?) the midline of the body. External rotation is turning (away from? toward?) the midline of the body.

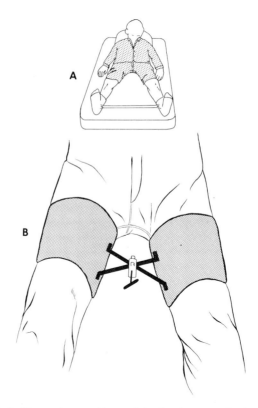

Fig. 11-4. A, Plaster boots with an abduction bar to maintain the position of the patient's legs. **B,** The position of the legs may also be maintained by placing a splint on the upper thighs.

64 If a cast or traction has not been applied, the nurse must utilize all available resources to maintain the patient's position. Sandbags and pillows can be placed alongside the operated limb and the patient's body to prevent movement and to serve as reminders. The

163

aspects of the hip surgery patient's position that need attention are:
a. The degree of flexion of the hip
b. The degree of abduction of the leg
c. The degree of rotation of the arm
d. The rotation of the leg

65 For other types of hip surgery these same aspects of the hip arthroplasty patient's position are regulated but to a lesser degree. Acute or sudden flexion of the hip joint must also be prevented after most hip arthroplasty procedures since it contributes to subluxation or dislocation of the operated joint. The major complications of hip surgery that can occur are joint _____

or _____ .

66 The aspects of the hip surgery patient's position to be controlled are _____ , _____ , and

_____ .

67 Abduction and external rotation of the operated leg can be maintained by using _____ ,

_____ , _____

_____ , and _____ .

68 Since the goals of medical and nursing care of the orthopedic patient are to assist the patient to maintain the function of the unaffected extremity and regain function of the affected part, complications related to inactivity or prolonged bed rest must not be permitted to develop. More attention is usually given to the operated leg and foot, but foot drop contractures can easily develop in both feet if adequate support is not provided. Three preventable musculo-

skeletal complications of hip surgery are _____ ,

_____ , and _____ .

69 External rotation contractures of the unoperated leg can occur if the patient remains in the same position in bed for an extended period of time. The sandbags and foot boards used to prevent foot drop also control the rotation of the leg. Two preventable postopera-

tive contractures are _____ and _____

_____ .

70 Once he is able to do so, the hip surgery patient often prefers to sit up in bed or in a chair because the sitting position is more easily attained than the side-lying position. If permitted to remain sitting for a long period, the patient may develop hip flexion contractures. Postoperatively, hip surgery patients may develop complications

related to _____ ,

_____ , and _____

_____ .

71 The nurse must concentrate efforts on preventing decubiti of the coccyx and other bony prominences. The patient's back must be rubbed with the appropriate substance or solution several times a day. Some factors that influence the development of decubiti in the elderly patient are:

a, b, and d

a. The patient's nutritional state
b. The turgor of the patient's skin
c. The patient's agility
d. The condition of the patient's skin before hospitalization

72 A sheepskin (real or synthetic) under the patient's back will help to keep it dry and thus prevent breakdown of the skin. The patient in traction may be helped by an alternating air pressure mattress. The bedridden patient may develop pressure sores on:

a, b, c, e, and f

a. The heel of the unoperated foot
b. The shoulder blades and spine
c. The coccyx
d. The knees
e. The elbows
f. Any bony prominence

73 If the patient is not in traction, he should be alternated between the supine and side-lying positions. The patient can be turned to the unoperated side as long as the prescribed rotation and abduction are retained. The patient who has had hip surgery is usually not

operated

turned to the _____ side.

74 The nurse should place pillows between the patient's legs if an abduction splint or spica cast is not in place. Of course, pillows must be placed between the lower legs and behind the patient's back to support him in the side-lying position. Pressure sores or decubiti are prevented by:

All of these

a. Massaging the skin over bony prominences
b. Turning the patient frequently
c. Using special pads and mattresses
d. Keeping the patient's skin clean and dry

75 The patient will require reassurance that turning will not disrupt the position of the hip joint. Smooth movements and adequate support can make turning a comfortable experience for the patient. Good nursing care of the postoperative hip surgery patient prevents

contractures; decubiti

the development of _____ and _____ .

165

76 Indicate which statements about the nursing care of the hip surgery patient are true and which are false.

True   _____ a. When turning the patient, the nurse supports the operated leg by placing the hands under the knee and the ankle.

False   _____ b. The obese elderly patient does not readily develop decubiti.

False   _____ c. When the patient is in traction, decubiti on the coccyx cannot be prevented.

True   _____ d. When an abduction splint is used, the operated leg still needs to be supported as the patient is turned.

77 Throughout the patient's postoperative convalescence, he must be encouraged to move and use his unaffected extremities as much as possible. The benefits of these movements include strengthening the arms in preparation for using crutches or a walker and prevention of thrombi. Exercise and movement of all extremities are essential to prevent _____ of the muscles.

atrophy

78 The patient should be taught to use the overbed trapeze and his unaffected leg to lift and move himself in bed. When he is in the correct sitting position, the patient's lungs can be completely expanded and aerated, and hypostatic pneumonia is prevented. The advantages of having the patient use an overbed trapeze are that:

a. He is able to assist in turning himself

b. His arms are strengthened

c. It facilitates nursing care

d. Movement helps to prevent complications

All of these

79 The patient who has hip surgery, whether it is a corrective procedure or an open reduction, is often elderly and not always in optimal physical condition prior to surgery. These patients quite frequently have medical conditions, such as arteriosclerosis and diabetes, for which adaptations in the nursing care plan must be made. A major nursing care goal for the patient who has had hip surgery is to _____.

prevent complications

80 There is no specific dietary prescription for the hip surgery patient, but an individualized nutritious diet should be provided. The patient's ability to chew as well as his preferences and needs should be considered. The nursing care plan is adapted according to:

a. The patient's medical condition

b. The type of surgery performed

c. The nurse's preferences

d. The patient's individual needs

a, b, and d

81 The patient who has had corrective hip surgery tends to know what to expect during his hospitalization. From the previous hospitalizations he has become accustomed to using the bedpan and no longer fears doing so, leaving inactivity and diet as the causes of constipation. Mr. Jones has had surgery on his right hip. When talking with him about his hip, the nurse should refer to it as his (right? bad? operated? game?) hip.

right or operated
(If you were unable to answer, review Sections one and two.)

82 Like most other postoperative orthopedic patients, the hip surgery patient experiences varying degrees of pain. Nursing care measures should be combined with the administration of analgesics to give the patient relief. Diversionary activities can be used to distract the patient from his pain and to encourage use of his hands and arms. Miss Brown is 76 years old and had left hip surgery 2 days ago. She has just asked the nurse to give her some linament to rub on her left hip. The nurse should:

b and d

a. Give her some linament
b. Change her position
c. Do nothing
d. Give her an analgesic

83 As the patient progresses, he will be permitted to sit up in a chair or to ambulate. The patient should be taught to pivot on the unoperated hip when getting out of bed. This method avoids trauma to the operated hip, which could be painful and could cause dislocation or subluxation of the hip. As the patient is being assisted from the bed to a chair, the possible complication that may occur is

dislocation or subluxation

_____.

As the patient sits in the chair, the possible complication that may develop is _____.

flexion contracture

84 List any six complications of hip surgery that can be prevented by good nursing care.

a. Hip flexion contractures
b. Decubiti
c. Hypostatic pneumonia
d. Thrombi
e. Dislocation of the hip
f. Subluxation of the hip
g. Foot drop
h. External rotation contractures
i. Constipation
j. Atrophy of muscles
(any six, any order)

a. _____
b. _____
c. _____
d. _____
e. _____
f. _____

85 Nursing measures used to prevent decubiti also make the patient more comfortable. List three nursing measures that contribute to the patient's comfort as well as prevent complications.

a. Using special pads or mattresses
b. Rubbing the patient's back
c. Supporting the affected limb

a. _____
_____
b. _____

d. Placing the patient on the unoperated hip when turning him or assisting him out of bed
(any three, any order)

c. _____

86 The physician performs an arthroplasty on the patient's hip joint because the patient has had continual stiffness and pain, which are the result of degenerative joint disease or old injuries. The arthroplasty operation:

a and b

a. Creates a joint that functions in the same manner as the former one
b. Creates a joint nearly like the original one
c. Is the ideal treatment for fractures

87 In an arthroplasty of the hip, the new joint can be created by replacement of the femoral head with prosthesis, by placement of some material between the joint surfaces (cup arthroplasty), or by replacement of both joint surfaces as is done in the total hip replacement procedure. The nurse must know which type of arthroplasty was performed in order to give the appropriate care. List the three types of hip arthroplasty procedures.

a. Cup arthroplasty
b. Femoral head prosthesis
c. Total hip replacement

a. _____
b. _____
c. _____

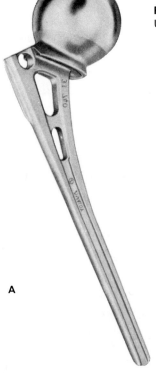
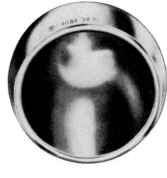

Fig. 11-5. **A,** Moore prosthesis. **B,** Femoral head cup. (Courtesy Zimmer • USA, Warsaw, Ind.)

A

B

88 The postoperative care of the patient who has had a cup arthroplasty differs somewhat from that of the patient who has had a prosthesis inserted or a total hip replacement. After a cup arthroplasty, the patient is placed in Russell's or balanced suspension traction, which supports the limb and helps maintain the prescribed degree of abduction and rotation. The indications for cup arthroplasty are:

a, c, and d
a. Degenerative joint disease
b. Fracture of the femur
c. Stiffness of the joint
d. Pain in the hip joint

89 The cup arthroplasty patient usually remains in traction for 2 to 3 weeks, during which time he should begin doing quadriceps-setting exercises. After the traction is removed, a more intensive exercise program should be instituted. Activities such as rocking in a rocking chair, pedaling a bicycle-like apparatus, and using a spring-controlled hip exerciser strengthen the muscles that control abduction, adduction, and flexion. While the patient is in traction, the nurse:

a, c, and d
a. Is responsible for applying traction principles
b. Supervises the patient as he does leg-raising exercises
c. Is responsible for preventing complications
d. Is responsible for making the patient comfortable

90 The cup arthroplasty patient is usually permitted to walk with crutches or a walker approximately 6 weeks after surgery, with no weight-bearing on the operated hip joint. The patient is taught to

unoperated
pivot on the _____ side.

91 The patient who has a femoral head prosthesis inserted may occasionally be placed in Russell's traction postoperatively, but he usually is permitted to be more mobile than the cup arthroplasty patient. The patient may be lifted into a chair soon after surgery and may walk with a walker a week or two later. The prosthesis pa-

can
tient (can? cannot?) be turned to the side-lying position.

92 Since the femoral head prosthesis patient's hip joint can be easily dislocated or subluxated, an abduction splint must be used at all times. Care must also be taken to prevent forced flexion of the hip. Are the following statements true or false?

True
_____ a. The cup arthroplasty patient does exercises to strengthen the muscles around the hip joint.

False
_____ b. Both the cup arthroplasty and femoral head prosthesis patient are routinely placed in traction.

False
_____ c. Balanced suspension traction after surgery is used to exert a gentle pulling force on the leg.

True
_____ d. Hip surgery patients are not permitted to bear

169

weight on the affected extremity when ambulating with a walker.

93 A total hip replacement procedure is performed when the hip joint has been extensively damaged by disease or injury, the patient has severe pain, or other forms of reconstructive surgery have not been successful or are not appropriate. Total hip replacement surgery is relatively new, and the ability of the prosthetic devices to withstand the stresses of walking and weight-bearing over an extended period of time (20 or 30 years) has not been proved. Therefore, surgeons tend to restrict its use to patients over 55 years old. The indications for the total hip replacement procedure are

extensive joint damage; severe pain; failure of other forms of surgery

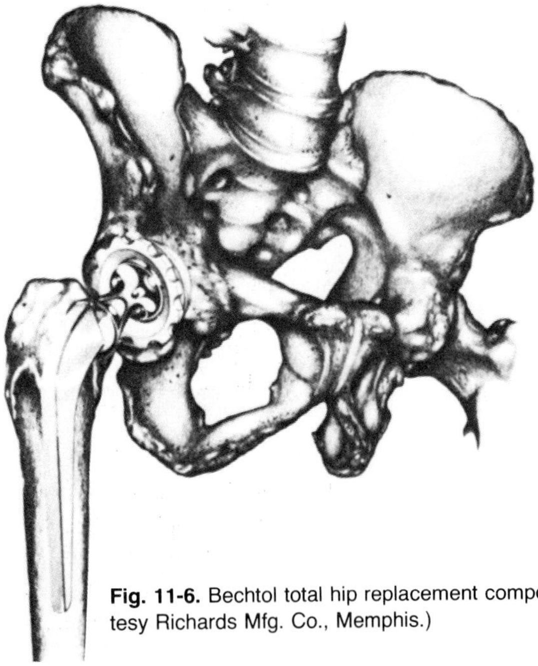

_____ , _____

_____ , and _____

_____ .

Fig. 11-6. Bechtol total hip replacement components. (Courtesy Richards Mfg. Co., Memphis.)

94 In the total hip replacement procedure, both surfaces of the patient's joint are replaced. A metal prosthesis is inserted in place of the head of the femur and a metal or polyethylene plastic cup replaces the acetabulum. Both devices are secured into position using methylmethacrylate, a cement. The total hip replacement procedure is a type of arthroplasty that can be described as being a combination

cup arthroplasty
femoral head prosthesis

of the _____

and _____

procedures. Total hip replacement is similar to a cup arthroplasty

an artificial acetabulum is inserted

because in both _____

_____ .

95 The preoperative preparation of the patient undergoing total hip replacement is essentially the same as that done for other patients. Preoperative nursing care of the patient includes _____ and _____ preparation and _____ _____ .

psychological
physical (skin); data collection

96 Laboratory studies are performed to confirm the preadmission diagnosis, to aid in diagnosing previously undetected or associated medical problems, and to provide baseline data for postoperative comparison. At the same time, blood samples may be taken for typing and cross-matching for replacement blood, which may be needed during or after surgery. If the physician requests that a preoperative prothrombin time be determined, it would suggest that postoperative treatment may include the administration of _____ .

anticoagulants

97 The physician may also request hip x-rays to be taken from various perspectives. These x-rays are utilized at the time of surgery to assist in the selection on the femoral prosthesis component. The x-rays provide information regarding femoral bone size and neck angle. Preoperative x-rays are used:

All of these

a. To assist in selection of prosthesis with appropriate femoral neck angle
b. To confirm extent of degenerative joint disease
c. To provide information about size of the medullary canal
d. To predict how successful the surgery will be in terms of improving joint range of motion

98 As was done with the total knee replacement patient, a dose of an antibiotic is frequently administered in the immediate preoperative period, in order to _____ .

prevent infection

99 Some surgeons have special operative skin preparation instructions. Some prefer that a depilatory be used rather than shaving the involved surgical site. In addition, the physician may request that the operative site be scrubbed with a bacteriostatic solution and that the area be covered with sterile linen just before the patient goes to surgery. These requests are made because research has shown that these measures do help to decrease the possibility of wound infection. A depilatory preparation may be preferred to shaving since shaving may abrade, nick, or cut the skin, creating a potential _____ _____ .

infection site

100 From the preceding discussion, it can be seen that one of the surgeon's primary concerns is _____ _____ .

prevention of infection

101 Preoperative instructions, demonstrations, and practice of postoperative exercises should occur while the patient is alert and cooperative. Quadriceps setting, gluteal setting, hula, and plantar and dorsiflexion foot exercises should be practiced before surgery. For the hula exercise, the patient pushes the foot on the affected side down as if to make the leg longer and then pulls it up as if to make the leg shorter. This exercise can be easily described by which of the following phrases?

b and c

a. Pull long
b. Push long
c. Pull short
d. Push short

102 Sit-ups with use of hand grips and a T-bar and hip hiking or posting should also be practiced preoperatively. These movements will facilitate nursing care and aid in the prevention of postoperative complications. When the patient chins himself on the T-bar the rib

atelectasis or hypostatic
pneumonia

cage fully expands and thus will help to prevent _____.

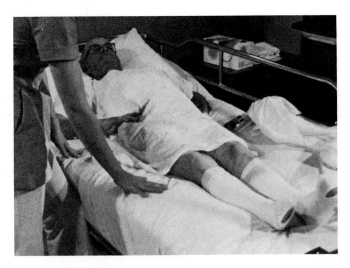

Fig. 11-7. For hula exercise, patient is instructed to alternately push long with foot and pull short with foot of the operative side. Note that this motion creates opposite position on unoperative side. (Courtesy Zimmer • USA, Warsaw, Ind.)

103 Sit-ups with the T-bar also contribute to the patient regaining mobility. Use of the T-bar contributes to strengthening of the arms

walking with a walker
or crutches

in preparation for _____.

172

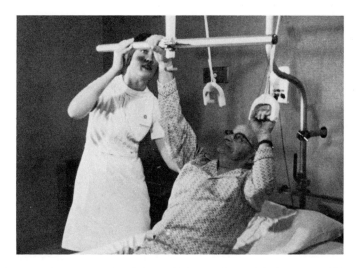

Fig. 11-8. Patient pulls himself up with hand grips and then moves to T-bar, where he can chin himself. (Courtesy Zimmer • USA, Warsaw, Ind.)

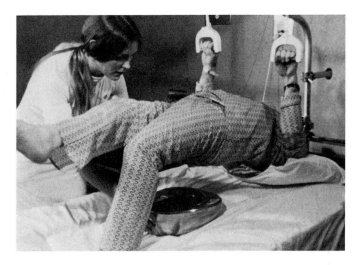

Fig. 11-9. Patient assumes post or hip hike position by grasping grips, arching head and neck into bed, and bringing opposite leg into deep flexion. Using opposite leg as a post to elevate body, operative hip and leg remain in a horizontal plane. (Courtesy Zimmer • USA, Warsaw, Ind.)

104 The hip hiking or post position facilitates nursing care without traumatizing the affected hip joint. The patient can assume this position while bed linen is being changed, while a bedpan is being placed under him, or while his back is being rubbed. List the exercises and movements that are taught to the total hip replacement patient preoperatively: _____

quadriceps and gluteal setting; plantar and dorsiflexion of foot; hula exercise; hip hiking; sit-ups with T-bar

_____ , _____

_____ , _____

_____ , _____ , and _____

_____ .

105 Some surgeons will request that the patient be placed in Russell's or Buck's traction postoperatively in order to maintain the allowed degree of abduction. When the use of traction is anticipated, the patient's bed, with the appropriate equipment attached, should be available in the operating room so the patient can be moved from the operating table into his bed. The physician usually makes the use of traction known as a part of his postoperative regimen. Before the
should patient goes to surgery, the purpose of the traction (should? should not?) be explained.

106 The nurse may also determine whether the patient will be using a walker or crutches postoperatively. Practice in their use should be a part of the total exercise program. The patient learns to
preoperatively walk with crutches _____ .

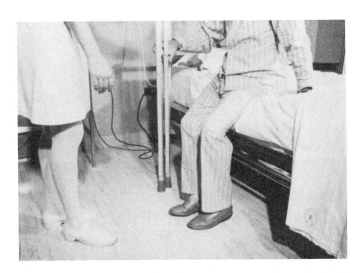

Fig. 11-10. Patient is taught to grasp his crutches together as a post, place them on operative side, and use them for support when ascending or descending. Opposite hand is then placed on bed. Patient maintains extension of affected leg while pulling himself up or letting himself down. (Courtesy Zimmer • USA, Warsaw, Ind.)

107 The total hip replacement surgical procedure is a major trauma to the body's physiological systems; therefore, the patient must be monitored closely for postoperative complications. Extensive blood loss during the surgical procedure from bleeding in deep soft tissues of the upper thigh as well as at the joint replacement sites should be anticipated. The nurse should observe the patient closely for indica-
hemorrhagic shock tions of _____ .

174

108 Observations for indications of shock include frequent measurement of vital signs, checking wound dressing and drainage, and measurement of hematocrit and hemoglobin levels. Evaluation of the observation is made by comparison with _____ _____ .

preoperative data

109 The surgeon may have inserted drains in the wound and connected them to mild suction. The drains facilitate observation and measurement of blood loss. If the patient is going into hemorrhagic shock, the nurse would notice that as the amount of drainage increased, the blood pressure _____ and the pulse rate _____ .

decreased

increased

110 The total hip replacement patient must be observed closely for indications of circulatory impairment and nerve damage. The potential peroneal nerve pressure points that must be checked when Russell's traction is in use are _____ _____ , and _____ , and _____ .

posterior aspect of knee; dorsum of foot; Achilles tendon
(If you were unable to answer, review Chapter 7.)

111 The circulation of the extremity in traction can be assessed by checking skin _____ and _____ , and by doing the _____ test.

color; temperature

blanching

112 An extensive list of "do's" and "don't's" for the postoperative total hip replacement patient could be compiled from the literature. The main theme throughout is to exercise to strengthen the muscles surrounding the hip joint so that flexion contractures can be prevented and/or corrected. Acute flexion of the hip must be avoided until the muscles are strong enough to hold the femoral head in the acetabulum. Abrupt, violent flexion of the hip joint can cause subluxation or dislocation of the femoral head prosthesis. The total hip replacement patient should avoid which of the following activities?

a. Sitting on a low stool
b. Squatting
c. Lying prone in bed
d. Climbing steep stairs
e. Crossing his legs at the knees

a, b, d, and e
(Lying prone is recommended to help prevent and/or correct hip flexion contractures.)

113 Thrombophlebitis and/or pulmonary emboli are complications of the total hip replacement procedure which must be prevented. Nursing actions which can be taken, in addition to administering the prescribed anticoagulant, include:

a. Encouraging patient to cough and deep breathe frequently
b. Instructing patient to chin self on T-bar

a, b, and d

c. Rubbing patient's legs with powder or lotion

d. Instructing patient to perform exercises

114 As long as the patient is receiving an anticoagulant, the nurse must monitor the patient for signs of _____, The nurse should be aware of the value of the _____ _____.

hemorrhage (bleeding)
prothrombin time

115 Some physicians prefer that the patient remain supine, while others permit turning of the patient onto the unoperated side (abduction must be maintained at all times). Pressure areas and decubiti are prevented by having the patient lift himself off the bed by hip hiking while back care is given. The affected leg must be maintained in _____ and _____.

abduction; extension

116 Progression of activities after total hip replacement is related to the condition of the wound—as the dressings and drain are removed from the wound, the patient can be more mobile. Nursing observations of the condition of the wound should include:

a, b, and c

a. Checking for sanguineous drainage

b. Checking for purulent drainage

c. Checking for skin approximation

d. Checking for proper placement of sutures

117 The most remarkable aspect of the total hip replacement patient's postoperative recovery is that he is permitted to ambulate with full weight-bearing on the affected extremity approximately 1 week after surgery. The patient uses a walker, crutches, or cane(s) for stability and experiences no pain when walking. Many of these patients have had severe hip pain for a number of years and are elated to be able to walk comfortably. Indicate which statements are true.

a and c

a. The nursing care of the hip surgery patient is adapted according to the procedure performed.

b. The nursing care of all hip surgery patients is the same.

c. The nursing care of the hip surgery patient is adapted to the patient's individual needs.

d. The postoperative recovery of all hip surgery patients proceeds at the same rate.

118 Infection is one of the most dreaded complications of total hip replacement surgery. Antibiotics are administered prophylactically, and precautions must be taken to prevent contamination of the wound. Infection is dreaded because _____ _____ _____ and _____ _____.

it may be necessary to remove the joint components; the patient may lose joint function

119 The first stage of treatment of an infected total hip includes open debridement of the wound with extensive irrigation with antibiotic solutions. Drains may be inserted in the wound to facilitate drainage or to permit continuous irrigation and suction. The initial, conservative approach to treatment of an infected total hip encompasses _____ _____ , _____ _____ _____ , _____ , and _____ .

debridement and irrigation of the wound; administration of intravenous and oral antibiotics; continuous irrigation; suction of the wound

120 When the conservative approach has not been successful, the prosthetic components and cement must be removed. The indications for removal of the components are continued pain and systemic manifestations of infection. Removal of the components requires the creation of a pseudarthrosis—a false joint—which is immobile. The disadvantages of a pseudarthrosis are instability and shortening of the limb. The prosthesis is removed when the patient _____ _____ _____ .

has continued pain and systemic infection

121 The removal of the prosthetic components is devastating for the patient who had anticipated pain-free full joint motion. The patient may have extreme difficulty accepting the loss of joint function and _____ and _____ _____ .

instability; shortening of the limb

122 The next most dreaded complication of total hip replacement surgery is loosening of one or both of the components. Pain associated with motion and weight-bearing is the cardinal sign of component loosening. The most serious complications of total hip replacement are _____ and _____ .

infection; loosening (of component(s)

123 At present, the only method of obtaining relief from pain is to remove the components and cement. This leads to development of a _____ .

pseudarthrosis

124 The pseudarthrosis is accompanied by lower limb _____ and _____ .

instability

shortening

125 The nurse is always alert for signs and symptoms of postoperative complications. The nurse observes the total hip replacement patient for signs of _____ , _____ , _____ , _____ , _____ _____ , _____ ,

subluxation; dislocation; flexion contractures; nerve damage; circulatory impairment; thrombophlebitis; hemorrhage (shock); infec-

tion; loosening of
component(s)

_____ , _____ , and
_____ .

126 The concept of total joint replacement is being extended; physicians have begun performing similar procedures on other joints. The basic concept of total joint replacement refers to:

b

a. Reconstruction of the joint with plastic surgery
b. Replacement of both articular surfaces
c. Insertion of a prosthesis

127 The osteotomy procedure is used to treat deformities and degenerative disease of the hip joint. An osteotomy is referred to as a

controlled fracture

_____ .

128 The arthrodesis procedure is sometimes the preferred procedure in the treatment of joint disease. When performing a cup arthroplasty, the physician revises the hip joint and inserts some material between the joint surfaces. If the physician does not insert a cup or other device, the joint would fuse together as it does in a(n)

arthrodesis

_____ .

129 The major disadvantage of an arthrodesis is that motion of the joint is permanently destroyed. The physician and patient must choose between joint pain and instability and joint motion. Joint motion is lost because the surgical procedure results in _____

joint fusion

_____ .

130 Arthrodesis and osteotomy patients are placed in a spica cast for 3 to 4 months after surgery to permit union. The purposes of the spica cast are:

a, c, and d

a. To immobilize the hip joint
b. To immobilize the patient
c. To maintain the degree of abduction
d. To facilitate nursing care of the patient

131 Which of the following should be incorporated in the nursing care plan of the patient who has just had a cup arthroplasty of the right hip and is in traction?

a, b, and d

a. Keep patient's bed clean and dry at all times
b. Check degree of flexion of patient's feet frequently
c. Place pillows behind patient's back when he is on his side
d. Encourage patient to use overbed trapeze to lift self

132 Which of the following should be incorporated in the nursing care plan of the patient who has a left hip prosthesis inserted?

a and d

a. Turn patient to right side or back only

b. Encourage patient to do his exercises

c. Remove abduction splint when patient is sitting in a chair

d. Lift patient into chair, maintaining abduction

133 Which of the following should be included in the nursing care plan of the patient who has a right total hip replacement?

a. Turn patient to left side or back only

b. Encourage patient to use T-bar to lift self

c. Maintain prescribed degree of abduction

d. Remind patient that he is not to put weight on right foot

134 After a cup arthroplasty, the patient is placed in _____ or _____ traction.

135 After a prosthesis has been inserted, the patient may be placed in _____ traction.

136 After a total hip replacement procedure has been performed, the patient may be placed in _____ or _____ traction.

137 An abduction splint is essential for the prosthesis patient because:

a. The prosthesis procedure is more extensive

b. The prosthesis can easily be broken

c. The prosthesis can easily be dislocated

d. The prosthesis can easily be subluxated

138 Russell's traction is applied after hip surgery in order to:

a. _____

b. _____

c. _____

139 Select the answer that is most correct. An arthrodesis can be performed on:

a. The knee and hip

b. The ankle and hip

c. The hip and shoulder

d. Any joint of the body

140 Three *major* goals of the nursing care plan for a patient having surgery of the lower extremity or hip are _____ _____, _____ _____, and _____ _____.

141 Both the patient in a spica cast and the patient who has had surgery on the lower extremity must be watched carefully for indications of _____ .

142 Which statement about the arthrodesis patient (ankle or hip) is correct?

a. There may be more complaints of pain after surgery.
b. The patient is allowed to ambulate with partial weight-bearing.
c. A large amount of wound drainage is not unusual.

143 The knee structures or parts most often injured are the _____ .

144 Immediately after removal of the menisci, the knee joint (may? may not?) be flexed.

145 The leg on which the meniscectomy was performed can be held in extension by using a _____ or a _____ .

146 Other purposes of the pressure dressing are to prevent _____ and _____ .

147 After knee surgery, the patient does _____ _____ , _____ , and _____ exercises.

148 Match the surgical procedure with the appropriate phrase.

_____ 1. Arthrodesis   a. Insertion of a prosthesis
_____ 2. Bunionectomy   b. Removal of a damaged part
_____ 3. Arthroplasty   c. Fusion of a joint
_____ 4. Meniscectomy   d. Removal of exostosis

149 The bunionectomy patient's feet are:

a. Checked frequently for bleeding
b. Elevated to prevent edema
c. Protected from trauma by a bed cradle
d. Positioned as the patient desires

150 The lower extremity and hip joint are used for _____ and _____ .

151 Which are common factors in the postoperative care of the patient who has had surgery on the lower extremity or hip joint?

a. The prevention of edema
b. The restriction of weight-bearing

c. The prevention of complications

d. The removal of growths

152 Mrs. Brown is a 60-year-old housewife who has a degenerative disease of the right hip joint. The surgical procedures that might be performed on her are a(n) _____, _____, _____, _____, or _____ _____.

cup arthroplasty; arthroplasty (prosthesis); arthrodesis; osteotomy; total hip replacement

153 Mrs. Brown has been admitted to the orthopedic unit and is to have a femoral head prosthesis inserted tomorrow. As a part of pre-operative teaching, the nurse tells Mrs. Brown:

a. She will be kept in bed for about a month

b. She may be in Russell's traction after surgery

c. She will need to use crutches or a walker when she begins walking after surgery

b and c

154 When Mrs. Brown is returned to her room after surgery, she is not placed in traction and the nurse checks the position of the patient's legs. They should be (adducted? abducted?).

abducted

155 The abduction must be maintained to prevent _____ or _____ of the hip joint (prosthesis).

dislocation

subluxation

156 Several hours after surgery, Mrs. Brown complains of pain in the operative site. After giving Mrs. Brown an analgesic, the nurse makes her more comfortable by _____ _____, _____, or _____.

changing her position; giving her back care; changing her bed linens; placing pillows to support her back and hips; raising or lowering the head and/or foot of the bed *(any three, any order)*

157 The nurse decides to turn Mrs. Brown. She can be turned to her _____ or her _____ side.

back; left (unoperated)

158 Two days after surgery the physician allows Mrs. Brown to sit up in a chair. Mrs. Brown is (walked to? lifted into?) the chair and her abduction splint is (left on? removed?).

lifted into

left on

159 Would either of the following necessitate changes in Mrs. Brown's care?

a. The development of postoperative complications

b. The presence of a medical condition such as heart disease

Yes

160 Mr. Brown has been admitted for a left total hip replacement.

181

infection

The preoperative skin preparation procedure has been altered to decrease the possibility of _____ .

quadriceps setting; hula;
   gluteal setting; plantar and
   dorsiflexion of the foot

161 Before Mr. Brown goes to surgery, the nurse instructs him in performing exercises such as _____

_____ , _____ , _____ ,

and _____

_____ .

crutches

walker; cane(s)

162 Mr. Brown may also practice ambulation with _____ ,

_____ , or _____ .

163 The nurse's initial assessment of Mr. Brown would include asking him questions about which of the following subjects?

All of these
(A—The nurse should
   evaluate the patient's needs
   for social services. B—Initi-
   ate consideration of discharge planning program.
   C—The nurse may need to
   clarify patient's perceptions.
   D—The nurse should
   identify history of past
   drug reactions.)

a. Financial resources

b. Living conditions at home

c. Expectations regarding the operative procedure

d. Medication taken in the past

164 Associate the terms in the left column with the related potential postoperative complications in the right column.

c

a, f

a, b, d

e

_____ 1. Prophylactic antibiotics   a. Thrombophlebitis

_____ 2. Anticoagulants   b. Dislocation

_____ 3. Exercises   c. Septic shock

_____ 4. Blanching test   d. Atelectasis

    e. Circulatory impairment

    f. Hemorrhage

instability

shortening

165 Pseudarthrosis is associated with lower limb _____

and _____ .

continuous
pain; systemic infection

pain on motion and
   weight-bearing

166 Infection of total joint replacement is indicated by _____

_____ and _____

_____ . Loosening of total joint replacements is indicated by _____

_____ .

the surgical procedure;
   administration of anesthesia; immobilization

167 Nursing care of the hip surgery patient is directed toward the prevention of complications that are related to _____

_____ , _____

_____ , and

_____ .

168 The function of the upper extremities is important when the patient has surgery on the lower extremities or hip joint because:

a. The patient may need to use crutches or a walker postoperatively
b. It contributes to the patient's overall ability to function postoperatively
c. The patient must be able to lift himself for back care to be given

169 In order to adequately plan and provide patient care, the nurse must:

a. Know how to prevent complications
b. Be able to identify the individual patient's problems
c. Know exactly how the procedure was performed
d. Be able to implement the appropriate nursing measures
e. Have a general understanding of the reasons for the procedure

170 The basic reasons for performing surgery on the hip joint are

joint _____ and/or _____ .

171 Surgery is performed on the lower extremity and hip joint to

permit the patient to bear weight and to walk _____
and _____ .

172 The factors influencing the nursing care of the orthopedic surgical patient are _____ ,

_____ , _____
_____ , and _____
_____ .

173 The main functions of the lower extremities and hip joints are

_____ and _____ .

174 Which of the following would be appropriate nursing goals for the patient who has had surgery of the lower extremity or hip joint?

a. To rehabilitate the patient
b. To assist the patient to resume functioning
c. To recognize the signs and symptoms of circulatory impairment
d. To prevent complications

175 On a separate page list the nursing care principles appropriate for the hip surgery patient and describe how you applied them when

caring for a patient.

CHAPTER 12

Principles of nursing care of the patient having surgery on the spine

1 Because of their erect posture, humans are prone to ailments of the low back, and low back pain is the most common complaint. Low back pain is caused by disease, accidental injuries, and poor body mechanics. Low back pain is a (symptom? disease?).

symptom

2 Low back pain is a symptom of arthritis of the spine, congenital spinal defects, tumors of the spine, infections of the spinal column, and a ruptured intervertebral disk. The onset of low back pain is often precipitated by trauma, such as a severe strain from lifting or a fall, or by repeated minor trauma from poor body mechanics. The disorders of the spine associated with low back pain include

arthritis; congenital defects; tumors; infections; ruptured disks

_____ , _____

_____ , _____ , _____ ,

and _____ .

3 The diagnosis of the exact cause of low back pain is often elusive. The physician utilizes the patient's history and physical examination, the nurse's assessment of the patient, laboratory tests, and roentgenograms to assist in determining the cause of the patient's low back pain. The nurse and physician obtain information from the patient about which of the following?

All of these
(Each aspect provides clues regarding injuries and body mechanics.)

a. Previous trauma

b. Occupation

c. Onset of pain

d. Avocational interests

4 Identification of the cause of the patient's low back pain is often further complicated by psychological problems. Since it is difficult to diagnose, low back pain is the ideal complaint for the hypochondriac, the malingerer, and the person who may desire some secondary gain from being disabled. To diagnose low back pain, the physician uses:

a, b, d, and e

a. Laboratory tests

b. The patient's history

c. Exploratory surgery

d. Roentgenograms

e. Physical examination

5 The nurse's assessment of the patient begins at the time of admission to the hospital and continues throughout his hospitalization. It is essential that the patient be assessed immediately so that the appropriate nursing measures may be instituted without delay if the patient is in acute distress. At the time of admission, the nurse observes the patient's posture for sciatic scoliosis, which is an involuntary protective mechanism the patient uses when the low back pain is associated with spinal nerve root irritation. The patient with sciatic scoliosis or listing appears to be leaning toward the side where there is spinal nerve root irritation. Sciatic scoliosis is a(n) (voluntary? involuntary?) response.

involuntary

6 The low back pain patient may also assume a posture of slight lumbar flexion, which makes the spine appear straight. The unaffected individual exhibits a lumbar lordosis, while the patient with low back pain may have _____.

lumbar flexion

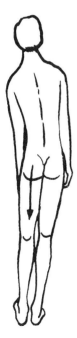

Fig. 12-1. Sciatic scoliosis. Patient with low back pain associated with spinal nerve root irritation appears to be leaning toward side of pain.

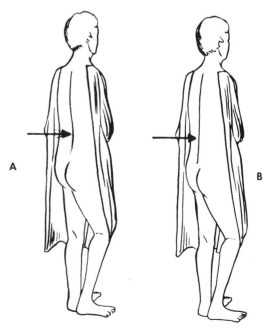

Fig. 12-2. A, Normal posture with slight lumbar lordosis or curvature at point of arrow. **B,** Flexion of spinal column; lordotic curve is no longer present.

185

7 At the time of admission the nurse observes the patient's posture

for _____ and _____

sciatic scoliosis; lumbar
flexion

_____ .

8 The nurse should assess the patient's pain in depth. The patient should be asked to describe the pain's onset, intensity, duration, location, and, if applicable, distribution. The low back pain patient with spinal nerve root involvement may have pain in the areas innervated by the irritated nerve. Knowledge of the pain's distribution assists the physician in determining the vertebral level of the nerve root(s) involved. The admitting nurse assesses the patient's

posture; pain

_____ and _____ .

9 The nurse begins the neuromuscular assessment by asking the patient to describe any paresthesia he may have. The patient may describe feelings of numbness, prickling, burning, tickling, or tingling. Knowledge of the pain assists the physician in determining the vertebral level of involvement. The nurse assesses the patient's

posture; pain; paresthesia

_____ , _____ , _____ .

sciatic scoliosis
lumbar flexion

10 The nurse checks the patient's posture for _____

_____ and _____ .

11 The nurse asks the patient to describe his pain in terms of its

onset; duration; intensity
location; distribution

_____ , _____ , _____ ,

_____ , and _____ .

vertebral level of spinal nerve
root involvement

12 Knowledge of pain and paresthesia distribution assist the physician in determining the _____

_____ .

13 Paresthesia is a general term referring to:

d

a. Increased sensitivity
b. Decreased sensitivity
c. Absence of sensation
d. Presence of a variety of sensations

numbness
prickling; burning
tickling; tingling

14 Paresthesia is defined as sensations of _____ ,

_____ , _____ ,

_____ , and/or _____ .

15 During the neuromuscular assessment, the nurse checks the patient for general extremity weakness, knee instability, foot drop, and muscle atrophy. The presence of these changes in an extremity indicates that the sensory and/or motor functions of the spinal nerve have been affected by the pathological process occurring in the spine. Changes in sensory and/or motor function of affected spinal

posture changes; pain;
paresthesia; extremity
weakness; knee instability;
foot drop; muscle atrophy

nerves are indicated by _____ ,
_____ , _____ , _____
_____ , _____
_____ , _____ , and _____
_____ .

16 The symptom of low back pain is very real to the patient, whether or not a cause can be found. The nurse must assume that all patients with low back pain have a legitimate reason for complaining until it is proved otherwise. While working with the patient with low back pain, the nurse sets a good example by (being pleasant? using good body mechanics? talking freely?).

using good body mechanics

17 The first goal of nursing care is to make the patient comfortable. The patient with low back pain has often been experiencing pain at home for days, weeks, or months and has experimented with numerous methods of relieving it. When the patient enters the hospital, he usually knows which measures are effective for him. (What is effective for one patient may be totally useless for another.) The nurse interacts with the patient to identify the nursing actions that can be used to assist him. The nurse identifies ways of meeting the patient's needs by _____
_____ .

using the interactive
nursing process

18 One or a combination of nursing measures may be utilized to make the patient more comfortable. The nursing measure that is helpful one day may be of no use the next day, so the nursing care plan must be reevaluated continuously and adapted on an individualized basis. The first goal of the nursing care plan for the patient with low back pain is to:
a. Assist the patient in accepting his diagnosis
b. Provide relief from symptoms
c. Determine the cause of the low back pain

b

19 Indicate which of the following statements are true and which are false.

False
_____ a. The nurse decides whether the patient really has a reason for low back pain or whether he is faking.

True
_____ b. Suggestions for means of making the patient more comfortable are elicited from the patient.

False
_____ c. Once a nursing measure is found to be helpful in relieving the pain, it will always be helpful.

True
_____ d. Combinations of various nursing care measures may provide relief from low back pain.

False   _____ e. The same nursing care measures are used for all patients with low back pain.

True   _____ f. The diagnosis of the exact cause of low back pain is difficult, and the physician uses many diagnostic tools to assist in making the diagnosis.

20 The spine must first be put at rest by placing the patient on a firm mattress, which supports the spine and legs. The orthopedic bed is made more firm by placing _____ under the mattress.

bedboards

21 The patient should be permitted to assume the position he finds most comfortable. The patient will usually lie on his side with his legs flexed or in William's position. Bedboards are placed on the patient's bed to _____.

support spine and legs

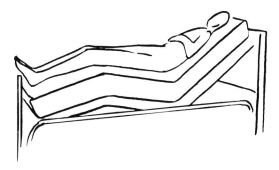

Fig. 12-3. In William's position, head of bed is elevated approximately 45 degrees, and flexed knees are supported by bed or pillows.

22 The William's position is comfortable for the low back pain patient because the lumbar lordosis is decreased and tension or pressure on spinal nerve roots may be diminished. The prone position is usually not comfortable for this patient and may be prohibited, since it might traumatize the spinal cord or spinal nerve. The positions most frequently assumed by the patient with low back pain are:

d and e

a. Lying on his back with his knees drawn up
b. Lying completely flat in bed
c. Lying on his right side
d. Lying on his side with his legs flexed
e. Lying in semi-Fowler's position with knees flexed

23 The patient may request or the nurse may suggest elevating the head of the bed and the portion of the bed under the knees. This position is known as _____.

William's position

Damage to the spinal cord and spinal nerves may be caused by lying in the _____ position.

prone

24 The nurse may administer analgesics and muscle relaxants, as prescribed, to help make the patient comfortable. At times, tranquilizers are also prescribed to help the patient adapt to being on bedrest. Administration of these medications and positioning the patient in bed are directed toward meeting the goal of _____

making the patient comfortable

———————————————————————————————————— .

25 Additional nursing care goals for the low back pain patient are to prepare the patient psychologically and physically for diagnostic procedures, promote mobility and independence, prepare the patient to resume activities of daily living, help the patient to accept physical limitations, help the patient to accept the treatment modality, and provide emotional support. These goals are necessary for the low back pain patient because the patient must accept and adapt to the conditions causing low back pain.

26 The degree and type of pain that the patient experiences vary with the individual and is affected by psychological factors. Which of these nursing measures are utilized when caring for the patient with low back pain?

b

a. Placing the patient in semi-Fowler's position
b. Talking with the patient and identifying those psychological problems contributing to his discomfort
c. Placing a small, firm pad under the supine patient's lumbar curvature
d. Placing the patient in prone position with bed flat

27 The physician may request that the patient be placed in pelvic, pelvic 90-90, or Buck's extension traction to reduce the lumbar lordosis. A side benefit is that being in traction requires that the patient remain in bed. The use of traction also decreases trauma to the spinal nerve root(s), which may in turn relieve painful muscle spasms. The patient in severe pain may need to become accustomed to the traction gradually. When pelvic and Buck's extension traction are used in the treatment of low back pain, the traction (must be continuous? may be intermittent?).

may be intermittent

28 The patient in severe pain can be helped to become accustomed to the traction by gradually increasing the amount of weight until the prescribed amount is comfortably tolerated. Alternately, the traction may be applied for a short time, removed for a while, and then replaced. Traction is used in the treatment of low back pain to

reduce lumbar lordosis

——————————————————————————————— .

29 When the patient is in pelvic traction, William's position may

The nurse gradually increases the amount of weight and alternately applies and removes the traction for short periods of time.

contribute to his comfort. Describe how the nurse helps the patient become accustomed to being in traction.

30 The application of moist heat to the lower lumbar region three or four times each day is very soothing and relaxing for some patients. Continuous applications of heat are not often employed since the constant heat may cause congestion of the tissues, thus aggravating the pain. Two measures that can be used to make the patient with low back pain more comfortable are _____ _____ and _____ _____ .

administering prescribed medications; changing patient's position; applying traction (Buck's, pelvic, or pelvic 90-90); applying moist heat *(any two, any order)*

may make the pain worse, may cause congestion

31 Massage of the lumbosacral area is sometimes beneficial, but other times this may stimulate muscle spasms. Continuous heat applications (soothe muscle spasms? may make the pain worse? may cause congestion? provide relief from pain?).

32 The administration of analgesics is combined with nursing care measures to enhance their effects. For example, after giving the analgesic, the nurse (should? should not?) rub the patient's back.

should, should not *(Both answers are correct; it depends upon the individual patient.)*

33 By discussing how to care for himself and what will be done to, for, or with him, the nurse conveys emotional support to the patient. Which of the following nursing actions would contribute toward meeting the identified nursing care goals?
a. Clarify patient's concept of the treatment
b. Describe use of heat, massage, and traction
c. Describe how to lift objects
d. Administer narcotic frequently to relieve pain

a, b, and c

34 The myelogram is a special x-ray technique utilized to identify obstructions of the spinal canal. X-rays are taken as a contrast material is injected into the subarachnoid space. The myelogram is used in conjunction with other information sources to identify the specific vertebral level of a spinal disease or condition where the pathology extends into the spinal canal. The myelogram is a (treatment? diagnostic?) procedure.

diagnostic

35 The nurse prepares the patient for a myelogram by:
a. Describing the procedure in terms he can understand
b. Presenting a lecture on the anatomy of the spine
c. Clarifying why the physician wants to perform the test

a and c

36 The indications for myelography include clinical evidence of a

190

protruding lumbar disk, possibility of a neoplasm, significant motor weakness from nerve root compression, and history of low back pain resulting from a ruptured disk that has not responded to conservative therapy and therefore the patient is a potential surgical candidate. A myelogram is performed

b

a. Routinely on all patients with low back pain
b. On selected patients to confirm a diagnosis
c. After surgery to assess results

37 A diskogram is performed to evaluate the disk pathology and confirm any nerve root trauma caused by disk disease or herniation. The myelogram shows the vertebral level of an obstruction of the spinal canal, while intervertebral disk disease is identified by

diskogram

_____ .

38 A diskogram is similar to the myelogram in that a contrast material is injected and x-rays are taken. However, in the diskogram, the contrast medium is injected into one or more specific intervertebral disks. Both procedures are somewhat hazardous and uncomfortable for the patient. Permanent damage to the spinal cord or any of the spinal nerve roots is extremely rare. The myelogram and

invasive

diskogram are (invasive? noninvasive?) procedures.

39 Diskography has not been generally accepted as a diagnostic procedure because it is somewhat painful and because there is a possibility that long-term untoward effects of inserting a needle into a normal disk may accelerate the normal degenerative changes of age and stress. A diskogram is performed:

c

a. Routinely on all low back pain patients
b. On selected patients to assess resulting surgery
c. To confirm a tentative diagnosis of intervertebral disk disease or condition

40 Electromyelographs will reveal evidence of motor changes secondary to nerve root involvement. Electromyelography is not a reliable indicator of muscle dysfunction until demyelinization has occurred (more than 3 weeks after onset of nerve root compression). The electromyelograph is one means of confirming a diagnosis. Intervertebral disk diseases and conditions may be identified by

physical examination; myelogram; diskogram; electromyelography

_____ ,
_____ , _____ , and
_____ .

41 After a myelogram, the physician aspirates the contrast media from the spinal canal. The physician may administer methylprednisolone acetate intrathecally to reduce possibility of postmyelogram

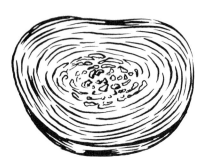

Fig. 12-4. Sectioned intervertebral disk with nucleus pulposus surrounded by annulus.

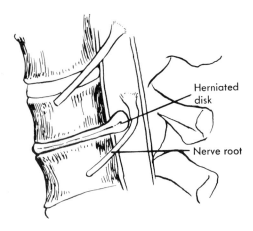

Herniated disk

Nerve root

Fig. 12-5. Nucleus pulposus ruptures annulus fibrosus and impinges on spinal nerve root.

discomfort and postspinal headache. Methylprednisolone acetate also helps to prevent inflammation of the spinal nerve roots (radiculitis). Possible postmyelogram complications are _____,

pain

spinal headache; radiculitis

_____ , and _____ .

42 The nurse instructs the postmyelogram patient to lie flat in bed and to drink large amounts of fluids. These actions help to prevent the development of postspinal headaches. Methylprednisolone acetate is administered intrathecally, which means it is injected into the

spinal canal

_____ .

43 Back pain may be found at any level of the spinal column since it is a symptom of a number of different diseases or conditions. Arthritis of the spine is a painful, disabling condition that affects many people. The arthritis may involve several vertebrae or a section of or the entire spinal column. Tumors, both benign and malignant, may also involve the spinal column, canal, or cord in some manner. Arthritis is discussed in general in a later section of this text; a discussion of tumors of the spine is beyond the scope of the text.

44 An intervertebral disk is a fibrocartilaginous retaining envelope for the fibrogelatinous nucleus pulposus, which is surrounded by the annulus fibrosus as shown in Fig. 12-4. The disks are located between each of the bony vertebrae of the spinal column. The nucleus pulposus may herniate through the annulus fibrosus and, depending on the direction of herniation, may impinge upon a nerve root, as shown in Fig. 12-5. The resultant irritation of the spinal nerve roots is referred to as radicular pain. Indicate which of the following statements is (are) true.

b and c

a. The only cause of low back pain is a slipped disk.

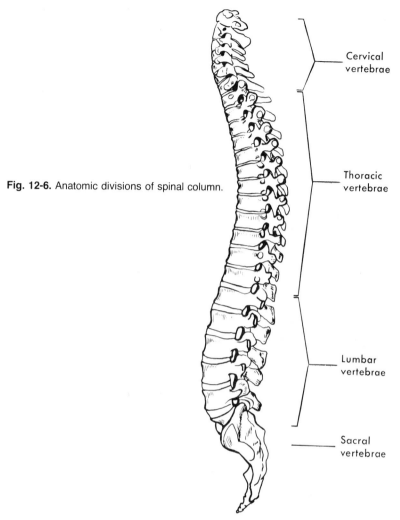

Fig. 12-6. Anatomic divisions of spinal column.

Cervical vertebrae

Thoracic vertebrae

Lumbar vertebrae

Sacral vertebrae

b. Arthritis of the spinal column may cause back pain.
c. A slipped disk is the same as a herniated nucleus pulposus.
d. Low back pain is a disease associated with trauma.

45 The most common intervertebral sites of herniation of the nucleus pulposus are L_4-L_5, L_5-S_1, C_5-C_6, and C_6-C_7. When the L_4-L_5 and the L_5-S_1 sites are involved, sciatic radiation of pain and/or paresthesia is a common sequela. The pattern of sciatic pain and paresthesia is radiation through the buttock and thigh, down the lateral aspect of the calf, and into the foot. The nurse assesses the patient's pain and paresthesia to aid the physician in identifying the

intervertebral site of herniation _____

_____ .

46 When the C_5-C_6 and C_6-C_7 intervertebral disks are herniated, the patient will experience shoulder and arm pain with numbness

193

and tingling in the hand and fingers. Sciatic radiation of pain and/or paresthesia is associated with herniation at the _____ and _____ levels.

L_4-L_5
L_5-S_1

47 Low back pain is often a symptom of an injury of the spinal region of the musculoskeletal system. Injuries to the spinal region are usually caused by

a, b, and d
(Heavy weights can be lifted without injury if proper lifting techniques are used.)

a. Improper lifting techniques
b. Accidental trauma
c. Lifting heavy weights
d. Poor body mechanics

48 Mr. Jones has had low back pain for 2 months because of a possible ruptured intervertebral disk and is currently extremely uncomfortable. The nurse:

b and d

a. Tells him that he should remain in the same position
b. Suggests that a warm moist pack be put on his back
c. Places a small firm pad under his lumbar curvature
d. Assists him to turn to a more comfortable position

49 Mr. Jones tells the nurse that at home he found that lying on his back on the floor and placing his legs on the seat of a chair was comfortable. He thinks that this would help him now. The nurse:

a and c

a. Acknowledges this as a good suggestion
b. Discourages him from using this position in the future
c. Assists him in attaining a similar position by lowering the head of his bed and sharply elevating the portion of the bed under his knees

50 To diagnose a ruptured intervertebral disk, the physician may request that a(n) _____ , _____ , or _____ be done.

myelogram; diskogram
electromyelogram

51 Loss of function may develop in the extremity supplied by the spinal nerve that is being irritated by the ruptured intervertebral disk. The nurse assesses the patient for loss of function by checking for _____ , _____ _____ , _____ , and _____ .

knee instability; foot drop;
extremity weakness;
muscle atrophy

52 When foot drop is detected on assessment, support must be provided for the affected foot to prevent the development of foot drop contractures. Foot drop contractures (can? cannot?) be corrected by exercising.

cannot

53 The nurse assesses the patient for problems associated with low back disorders, plans nursing care based on the assessment, implements the planned actions, and reevaluates the patient to ascertain the impact of nursing care. Indicate which statement(s) is (are) true.

b and c

a. The nursing process can be applied only when caring for surgical patients.
b. The nursing process is composed of four basic phases—assess, plan, implement, and evaluate.
c. The nursing process is applicable in all health care situations.

54 A herniated nucleus pulposus or ruptured intervertebral disk, as it is also known, is the most common cause of low back pain. The symptoms of a ruptured intervertebral disk include which of the following?

a, b, and d

a. Radiating leg pain
b. Paresthesia of the foot
c. Gluteal region spasms
d. Gluteal region pain

55 Stenosis or narrowing of the spinal canal in the cervical and lumbar region has been detected more often in recent years than it had been in the past, because of improved diagnostic techniques. Stenotic lumbar spinal canal is often observed with a herniated lumbar disk or spondylosis. Lumbar spinal stenosis may be congenital but symptoms are more often seen after the age of 35. Spinal stenosis

narrowing

is _____ of the spinal canal.

56 The patient with lumbar spinal stenosis often has radiating pain because the nerve roots on one or both sides are involved. Radiating pain from compressed spinal nerve roots is referred to as

radicular

_____ pain.

57 The bed position of comfort for the stenotic patient is usually a semi-Fowler's position with the hips and knees flexed. The patient's posture is somewhat abnormal in that he is more comfortable bending forward, which produces flexion of the normal lordotic curve.

is not

Lumbar spinal stenosis (is? is not?) caused by a ruptured disk.

58 The nurse can help the lumbar spinal stenosis patient by changing his bed position to _____

semi-Fowler's position with hips and knees flexed

_____ .

59 Spinal stenosis and herniated nucleus pulposus are usually treated conservatively with bedrest, medication, and traction.

60 *Laminectomy* is the removal of a portion of the lamina of one or

195

more vertebrae and the portion of the nucleus pulposus that is protruding or ruptured from the intervertebral disk. A laminectomy is:

a. Performed as treatment for arthritis
b. The removal of protruding nucleus pulposus
c. The removal of part of the vertebral lamina
d. Usually performed after conservative therapy has been unsuccessful

61 *Spinal fusion* is an arthrodesis of one or more vertebrae of the spine. Fusion of the vertebrae is obtained by placing a piece of bone from elsewhere in the body over the area of the vertebrae where fusion is desired. A spinal fusion is a(n) (arthrotomy? arthroplasty? arthrodesis? laminectomy?).

62 Laminectomy may be done by itself or combined with spinal fusion for effective treatment of ruptured intervertebral disks. Spinal fusions without laminectomy are performed to prevent or correct deformities or to stabilize a spine weakened by disease. Indicate whether the following statements are true or false.

_____ a. The physician performs a laminectomy on the patient with arthritis of the spine to remove the diseased part.

_____ b. The physician performs a laminectomy and spinal fusion to remove a protruding nucleus pulposus and to perform an arthrodesis of the vertebrae.

63 The preoperative preparation of the patient having surgery on the spine is essentially the same as that of other orthopedic patients. The nurse must know which procedure the surgeon plans to do so that

the patient's skin can be properly prepared by _____

_____

and _____

_____ .

64 The skin over the bone graft donor site must also be prepared when a spinal fusion is planned. Either the iliac crest or the anterior tibia is the usual donor site. The bone graft (replaces the removed

vertebral arch? is placed over the vertebrae where fusion is desired?).

65 During the surgical procedure the spinal cord, spinal nerves, and blood vessels may be traumatized. The nurse therefore observes the postoperative patient closely for indications of hemorrhage and nerve damage. The nurse monitors the patient's ability to move his feet and legs, the presence of sensation below the operative site, and the functioning of the patient's bowels and bladder. Two possible compli-

cations of back surgery are _____ and

_____ .

66 The nurse should ask the patient to move his feet and legs and watch as he does so. If the patient is not able to do this, it could be an indication of damage to the _____ or _____ .

spinal cord
spinal nerves

67 The nurse touches the patient's feet and legs in order to test _____ .

patient's ability to feel
(sensation)

68 The indications of postoperative nerve damage are loss of _____ , _____ , and _____ .

motion; sensation
bowel or bladder function

69 Although there may be no damage, the tone of the bladder and bowels may be diminished from the trauma of the surgical procedure. If an indwelling catheter has not been inserted, the patient should feel the need to urinate several hours after surgery and should be able to empty his bladder completely. After laminectomy and/or spinal fusion, the nurse observes the patient for complications by:
a. Asking him if he can tell whether the nurse has a hand on his foot
b. Asking the patient to move his feet
c. Asking the patient if he feels the need to urinate
d. Asking the patient to move his hands and arms

a, b, and c
(d would be correct if the
patient had surgery on
cervical vertebrae.)

70 Soon after surgery, the patient's bowels should resume normal activity. Along with a loss of bowel tone, the _____ may be diminished.

bladder tone

71 The physician may prefer that the patient be placed in the supine position during the immediate postoperative period to retard hematoma formation. The side-lying position facilitates inspection of the surgical dressing and is safer for the waking patient. The laminectomy and spinal fusion patient is watched closely for signs of _____ or _____ .

nerve damage; hemorrhage

72 Although a spinal fusion is like an arthrodesis in other respects, there should be no drainage or bleeding evident on the surgical dressing. Indications of hemorrhage are:
a. Decreased pulse rate
b. Decreased blood pressure
c. Evidence of active bleeding (drainage)
d. Increased pulse rate

b, c, and d

73 The indications of spinal cord or spinal nerve damage or trauma are:
a. Patient is unable to move his feet or legs
b. Patient feels no urge to urinate when his bladder is palpable

a, b, and d

c. Patient has large amount of sanguineous drainage on dressing

d. Patient cannot tell when nurse places a hand on his foot

74 The physician usually permits the patient to be turned postoperatively; the patient's body must be kept in one plane as he is moved. Until the patient is able to assist, the nurse should have another member of the staff assist. The patient's position after surgery is determined by:

b, c, and d

a. The patient's preference

b. The type of surgery performed

c. The patient's degree of alertness

d. The physician's preference

75 To keep the patient's body in one plane while turning him (which prevents trauma to the graft site and incision), the nurse rolls him as if he were a log. A folded sheet placed under the patient's torso is very helpful. If the patient is to be "log-rolled":

b, c, and d

a. His hips are turned first, followed by his shoulders

b. The nurse must have assistance—either the patient, another staff member, or a turning sheet

c. The patient's hips and shoulders are moved at the same time, with no twisting action on the spine

d. The nurse teaches the patient to "log-roll" if he is sufficiently alert

76 The spinal surgery patient is "log-rolled" in order to prevent

trauma to the graft site or incision

_____

_____ .

77 The patient who has had a laminectomy, without fusion, is usually permitted to ambulate soon after surgery. Early ambulation aids in the prevention of postoperative complications such as

atelectasis; hypostatic pneumonia; decubiti; thrombophlebitis; pulmonary emboli; muscle atrophy; contractures

_____ , _____

_____ , _____ , _____

_____ , _____ ,

_____ , and _____ .

78 The patient who has had a spinal fusion may not be permitted to get out of bed until a week or two after surgery. While the patient is confined to bed, measures must be taken to prevent foot drop and external rotation contractures. Contractures are prevented by using

sandbags; foot boards; pillows or other devices (any two, any order)

supportive devices such as _____

and _____ .

79 The postoperative nursing care of the spinal surgery patient is

recognition; prevention

directed toward _____ and _____ of complications.

80 While the patient is in bed, the bed must remain flat, but pillows can be placed under the knees or lower legs for comfort. The "log-rolling" technique is used to:

b

a. Keep the patient flat in bed
b. Maintain the hips and shoulders in one plane
c. Prevent trauma to the arms and legs

81 The spinal fusion patient must be taught to continue to "log-roll" until complete union of the graft has occurred. If the spinal

may not

surgery patient requests it, the head of his bed (may? may not?) be elevated.

82 The patient who has had a spinal fusion is not permitted to ambulate without a corset or brace. The corset or brace must be fitted by someone knowledgeable in the technique. When he is up, the

is not

laminectomy patient (is? is not?) required to wear a brace. When he

is

is up, the spinal fusion patient (is? is not?) required to wear a brace.

83 The corset or brace must be put on while the patient is in the supine position. The patient should be instructed to follow the same procedure when putting the brace on by himself. The corset or

sitting in a chair;
walking around; sitting
on the toilet

brace is worn by the patient when (sitting in a chair? walking around? sitting on the toilet? lying in bed?).

84 A body cast or plaster jacket may be necessary if the spinal fusion was done to correct a deformity. The plaster cast maintains the corrected position until union has occurred. Indicate which statements are true and which are false.

False

_____ a. All laminectomy patients must wear a brace after surgery.

True

_____ b. The spinal fusion patient must wear a corset or brace whenever he is not in bed.

True

_____ c. The patient who has had a corrective spinal fusion may have a plaster cast applied postoperatively.

False

_____ d. All spinal surgery patients must wear a supportive device.

arthrodesis

85 A spinal fusion is a(n) _____ of one or

vertebrae

more _____ .

lamina

86 A laminectomy is the removal of part of the _____

herniated nucleus pulposus

and _____ .

are not

87 A laminectomy and spinal fusion (are? are not?) always done together.

199

88 Which statement is true?

a. The patient can have a laminectomy done and not a spinal fusion.

b. The patient cannot have a spinal fusion done without a laminectomy.

89 The most prevalent symptom of a spinal disease or condition is _____ .

90 Low back pain is a symptom of _____

_____ , _____

_____ , _____ , _____

_____ , _____

_____ , and/or _____

_____ .

91 Three special diagnostic procedures used to identify or confirm the cause of back pain are _____ , _____ , and _____ .

92 Which of the following are potential complications of myelogram?

a. Radicular pain

b. Spinal headache

c. Transient paralysis

d. Permanent paralysis

93 Nursing actions which can be taken to prevent postspinal headache after a myelogram include _____ _____ and _____ _____ .

94 A diskogram will show any defects, disease, or disruption of a(n) _____ .

95 Diskograms are not routinely done by all physicians because _____ _____ _____ _____ .

96 On admission, the nurse assesses the low back pain patient's _____ , _____ , and _____ .

97 The low back pain patient may involuntarily change his posture so that he has _____ and/or _____ .

98 The nurse asks the low back pain patient to describe his pain in terms of its _____ , _____ , _____ , _____ , and _____ .

onset; intensity; duration
location; distribution

99 Knowing the distribution of pain and paresthesia provides clues as to the _____
_____ .

vertebral level of the nerve
root involvement

100 When the patient has a herniated nucleus pulposus in the cervical spine, the pain usually will radiate _____
_____
_____ .

through the shoulder and arm
and down to the hand and
fingers of the affected side

101 Why is it important to be familiar with the abdominal vascular anatomy when the patient has had a lumbar laminectomy?

Knowing that the abdominal
aorta lies close to the spine
suggests that hemorrhage
may be a complication of
lumbar laminectomy.

102 The basics of conservative management of the patient with a ruptured intervertebral disk are _____ , _____ , and _____ .

bedrest; medications (analgesics, muscle relaxants,
and tranquilizers); traction

103 The types of traction used in the treatment of low back pain include _____ , _____ , and _____
_____ .

Buck's; pelvic; pelvic
90-90

104 The type of traction used in the treatment of a ruptured intervertebral disk in the neck is _____ .

cervical traction
(Refer to Chapter 8.)

105 The nursing care plan for the patient with low back pain is:
a. Predetermined and rigidly enforced
b. Designed to meet the individual's needs
c. Adapted as the patient's responses change
d. Structured for continuous use without change

b and c

106 The nursing care plan for the patient with low back pain should be designed to meet his _____ and _____ needs.

physical; psychological

107 Mr. Brown enters the hospital complaining of low back pain. Number the steps of his diagnosis and treatment in the order of their probable occurrence.

4 _____ Perform myelogram
3 _____ Place patient in traction
5 _____ Perform laminectomy
1 _____ Place patient on bed rest
2 _____ Obtain history and laboratory examinations

108 A myelogram is:

a. An x-ray technique used to diagnose arthritis of the spine
b. An x-ray technique used to identify a ruptured vertebral arch
c. An x-ray procedure used to identify tumors of the spine
d. An x-ray technique that the physician utilizes in diagnosing a ruptured disk

109 Three nursing actions used to make the patient with low back pain more comfortable are _____

_____ ,

_____

_____ , and

_____

_____ .

110 List two positions which the patient with low back pain might find comfortable.

a. _____

b. _____

111 How can the patient in severe pain be assisted in becoming adjusted to pelvic traction?

a. _____

_____

b. _____

_____

112 Proper body mechanics include using the correct posture when sitting in a chair. A straight-backed, firm chair is best suited for maintaining the correct posture. It is essential that the low back pain patient maintain the correct posture since this will prevent or reduce radicular pain. The hospital bed is prepared for the low back pain patient by _____

_____ .

113 Analgesics and/or muscle relaxants are usually prescribed on an as-needed basis for the low back pain patient. The patient should be instructed to request medication before the pain becomes severe. Other means of relieving pain are _____ , _____ ,

_____ , and

_____ .

114 Maintaining bedrest is an important factor in controlling back pain when the patient has spinal stenosis or a ruptured disk. Usually, the patient is permitted to walk to the bathroom because using a bedpan is very uncomfortable. Throughout his hospital stay the patient is taught to use good body mechanics, including correct

posture

_____ .

115 Good body mechanics includes using the proper lifting techniques. The low back pain patient should *not* use an overbed trapeze or similar self-help devices since he might use his back muscles inappropriately and thus generate tension on the spine or stimulate painful muscle spasms. However, the patient can use bed siderails when they are up to help turn himself. Good body mechanics includes assuming the correct posture when (sitting? standing? lifting? lying in bed? turning?).

All of these

116 The low back pain patient should be instructed not to get out of bed without assistance and to use a walker or cane if he has severe leg involvement. These safety measures should be implemented to protect the patient from accidental injury. A planned patient teaching program should include instructions regarding _____

body mechanics; activity limitations; safety measures

_____ , _____

_____ , and _____ .

117 Muscle spasms may be triggered by irritation of the spinal nerves or may be associated with lumbosacral strain. Lumbosacral muscle strain may be the result of poor lifting techniques or direct trauma to the back. Bedrest, medication, and physiotherapy will usually bring about improvement. Continued poor posture or improper body mechanics can lead to chronic lumbosacral strain. Low back problems, whether manifested by severe muscle spasms or by severe pain, may be caused by (accidental injury? poor body mechanics? disease? congenital defect?)

All of these

118 A herniated nucleus pulposus may be treated by injecting it with a diskolytic substance such as chymopapain. The chymopapain is injected into the intervertebral disk while the patient is under general anesthesia. This method of treatment is still under investigation and is not in general use because the results have not been totally satisfactory. At this time the numerous potential complications and the unreliable results restrict its use.

119 Match the diagnosis with the surgical procedure used for treatment.

a and/or b
b
b

_____ 1. Ruptured intervertebral disk   a. Laminectomy
_____ 2. Congenital spinal deformity   b. Spinal fusion
_____ 3. Arthritis of the spine

120 The postoperative patient should be watched closely for indica-

nerve damage; hemorrhage

tions of _____ and _____ .

121 Describe briefly how the postoperative patient is moved in bed.

122 The nurse detects indications of postoperative nerve damage by:
a. Asking the patient how his feet feel
b. Asking the patient if he can tell when his bladder is full
c. Doing the blanching test on his toes
d. Asking the patient to move his feet

123 If the patient has had a laminectomy to remove a ruptured intervertebral disk:
a. His preoperative radiating leg pain will no longer be felt
b. His preoperative leg pain may continue postoperatively
c. His radiating leg pain is an indication of surgical trauma

124 Postoperatively, the nurse must teach the spinal fusion patient _____ and

_____

_____ .

125 Postoperatively, the spinal fusion patient wears a brace or corset (when) _____ .

126 Low back pain is a (symptom? diagnosis?).

127 Mr. Jones is a 45-year-old laborer, is married, and has five children. He has been admitted to the orthopedic unit and is complaining of low back pain. His pain may be a symptom of a(n)

_____ ,

_____ ,

_____ , _____ ,

_____

_____ , _____

_____ , or _____ .

128 List three objectives of Mr. Jones' nursing care plan.

a. _____

_____

b. _____

_____

c. _____

_____

129 The physician has requested that a myelogram be performed on Mr. Jones to see if he has a _____
_____.

tumor or ruptured intervertebral disk

130 After his myelogram, the nurse tells Mr. Jones to _____
_____,
and to _____
_____.

lie flat in bed for 24 hours; drink copious amounts of fluids

131 The nurse has instructed Mr. Jones to do these activities in order to prevent _____
_____.

a postmyelogram headache or radiculitis

132 The physician has left orders for Mr. Jones to be prepared for surgery. Mr. Jones is to have a spinal fusion done; the possible bone graft donor sites are his _____
or _____.

anterior tibia (right or left)
iliac crest (right or left)

133 The physician has performed a laminectomy and spinal fusion on Mr. Jones. Postoperatively, the nurse checks him for indications of nerve damage. The indications that this complication has occurred are:

a. Loss of extremity motion
b. Loss of sensation
c. Decreased bladder or bowel tone

a. _____
b. _____
c. _____

134 The nurse is turning Mr. Jones for the first time since surgery. He can be log-rolled easily if she _____
_____ or _____
_____.

uses a turning sheet
has adequate assistance

135 Mr. Jones is unable to move his legs, which is an indication of:
a. Surgical trauma to the blood vessels
b. Possible surgical trauma to the spinal cord or spinal nerves
c. Surgical trauma to the spinal nerves and vessels

b

136 Mr. Jones does not have an indwelling catheter. Therefore, the nurse checks his ability to void because his _____
may be diminished.

bladder tone

137 Mr. Jones will be permitted to be up walking around:
a. In a day or so
b. With his brace on
c. With his plaster jacket on

b

138 Mr. Jones wants to return to his former job after discharge from his physician's care. The physician will probably approve of his doing so if Mr. Jones (becomes a nonworking supervisor? learns body mechanics that will prevent future injury?).

learns body mechanics that will prevent future injury

139 Two postoperative complications that can be prevented by good nursing care are _____ and _____ .

foot drop

external rotation contractures

140 The physician may have difficulty diagnosing the patient's low back pain because:

a. _____
_____
b. _____
_____

a. There are many causes for low back pain.
b. The patient's psychological problems may intervene.

141 Complaints of low back pain would not be so prevalent if:

a. People practiced good body mechanics
b. People would put their backs "into it" when they lift things
c. People walked on all four limbs instead of two

a and c

142 The nursing care plan for the patient with low back pain is developed:

a. By the nurse(s) and the patient
b. For the patient by the nursing team
c. On basis of nurse-patient interactions
d. With the intention that it will not change

a and c

143 The primary aim of nursing care of the patient with low back pain to assist him to resume normal functioning. On a separate piece of paper write the nursing care plan that you developed to lead to attainment of this aim for the following types of patients you have cared for:

a. A patient who is receiving conservative therapy for low back pain and will not be having surgery
b. A patient who has had a laminectomy and spinal fusion as treatment for a ruptured intervertebral disk

Discuss your care plans with your instructor and/or discuss your care plans in class. Specifically, discuss how the plan was adapted as the patient's needs changed.

CHAPTER 13

Principles of nursing care of the amputee

1 There are numerous medical and surgical conditions for which the treatment necessitates removal of all or a portion of an extremity. For example, the surgeon may amputate the patient's entire leg via disarticulation at the hip joint or may remove only the part below the knee. To amputate is to _____

_____ .

surgically remove all or a
portion of an extremity

2 The conditions that may require an amputation include peripheral vascular insufficiency, peripheral vasospastic disease, trauma, malignant and benign tumors, chronic infections, thermal injury, and miscellaneous conditions such as gas gangrene of the extremity. Amputation after trauma may be necessary to remove a severely damaged portion of an extremity or to create a functional stump when the traumatic amputation has been complete. Amputation may be indicated when the patient has:

a, c, d, and e

a. Tissue necrosis caused by frostbite
b. Thrombophlebitis
c. Mangled hand
d. Arteriosclerosis involving an extremity
e. Raynaud's disease

3 The portion of the extremity that remains after the surgical amputation is the *stump,* and the patient who has had an amputation is referred to as an *amputee.* Which part (A or B) of the leg shown in Fig. 13-1 will be the stump? _____

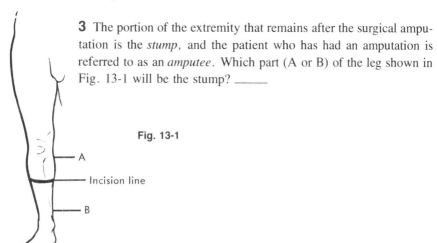

Fig. 13-1

A

Incision line

B

4 The surgical approach to amputation varies with the underlying indication for amputation. When the lower extremity is involved, the surgeon's goal is to create a weight-bearing stump. The surgeon may remove the bone and suture the skin flaps over the end of the bone, as shown in Fig. 13-2, *A* and *B*. This approach forms a *closed* amputation, with the anterior flap coming around to cover the end of the bone and with the suture line posterior to the portion of the stump that will bear weight. In a closed amputation the skin flaps (do? do not?) cover the end of the bone and the suture line (will? will not?) be in a position to bear weight.

do
will not

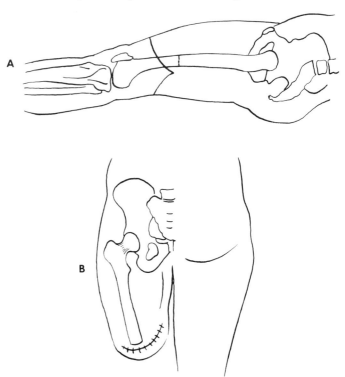

Fig. 13-2. A, Above the knee closed amputation; bone incision line indicated by line transecting the bone. **B,** Stump of closed amputation; suture line located posteriorly.

5 When the patient has had an infection, the skin flaps may not be sutured closed over the stump end so that the wound can drain freely. An *open* amputation is shown in Fig. 13-3. The skin flaps are sutured in a(n) (open? closed?) amputation.

closed

6 When the affected extremity is infected, the surgeon may amputate the extremity without creating flaps to cover the end of the bone, as shown in Fig. 13-4. After a guillotine amputation, the wound is approximated via skin traction or secondary closure to complete the

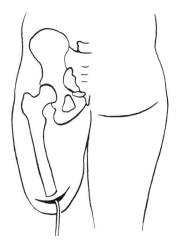

Fig. 13-3. Open amputation of leg (above knee) with drain in place.

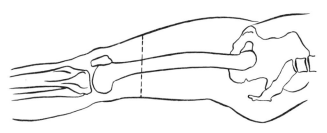

Fig. 13-4. Guillotine amputation of lower leg; incision line indicated by broken line.

open; closed; guillotine

stump. The types of amputations which may be performed are _____ , _____ , and _____ .

7 The principles of preoperative nursing care are generally applicable in the care of patients who are having an amputation performed. However, more emphasis is placed on the psychological preparation of the patient, since the patient needs to be assured that, after surgery, normal activity can be resumed by using a prosthesis fitted to the stump. In other words, the preoperative nursing care of the patient having an amputation focuses on the same primary goal as other aspects of orthopedic nursing. The *primary goal* of orthopedic nursing is to assist the patient:

c

a. To maintain meaningful family relationships
b. To accept his diagnosis
c. To regain normal function
d. In identifying appropriate coping mechanisms

8 The psychological preparation of the surgical patient is the first phase of rehabilitation. However, when the amputation is associated with trauma there may not be any opportunity for preoperative psychological preparation. Upper extremity amputations are often traumatic and psychological preparation for these patients is, for the most part, precluded. When does the rehabilitation process usually start for the amputee? _____

preoperatively

9 The psychological preparation should be such that the patient is permitted to progress through the stages of the grieving process. The amputee can be expected to grieve over the anticipated or actual loss of a limb similar to the grieving associated with death. When the patient is scheduled to have an amputation, the nurse should prepare the patient psychologically by _____
_____ .

assisting the patient in the grieving process

10 The physical preparation of the patient should include an exercise program when possible. Preoperatively the patient having an above-the-knee (AK) or a below-the-knee (BK) amputation should be taught and should practice gluteal and quadriceps setting and range of motion exercises. Range of motion exercises of the upper extremity are also indicated preoperatively. The preoperative preparation of the amputee includes _____ and _____ elements.

psychological
physical

11 The patient scheduled for a below-the-knee amputation should perform _____ , _____
_____ , and _____
_____ exercises.

gluteal setting; quadriceps setting; range of motion

12 As in preoperative care, the principles of postoperative nursing care are generally applicable in the postoperative care of an amputee. When a limb is amputated, major blood vessels are surgically severed. Therefore, an amputation presents a greater potential for postoperative hemorrhage than do many other procedures, and the nurse must observe the patient closely. Hemorrhage is more likely to occur after amputation because (major blood vessels? bones and tissues?) have been cut.

major blood vessels

13 Signs of hemorrhage and impending shock include a lowered blood pressure, a rapid, thready pulse, and loss of blood. Postoperatively, the nurse should check the patient's blood pressure, pulse, and dressings frequently for signs of _____ .

hemorrhage

14 The signs of hemorrhage that the nurse should watch for are
_____ ,
_____ ,
and _____ .

lowered blood pressure
rapid, thready pulse
loss of blood

210

15 If the wound becomes infected, postoperative hemorrhage may be caused by necrosis of a blood vessel. Because of the gravitational flow, wound drainage is often found beneath the stump; therefore, the nurse must remember to examine the (underside? edges?) of the stump dressing.

underside

16 If signs of hemorrhage are present in an above- or below-the-knee amputation, the nurse should elevate the foot of the patient's bed, not the stump. In addition to reporting the observation to the physician, what can the nurse do when signs of hemorrhage are present?

Elevate the foot of the bed.

17 The physician may request that a tourniquet be kept at the bedside for use if the patient's stump begins hemorrhaging. However, tourniquets are used only in cases of severe hemorrhage, because direct hand pressure is usually adequate. Why is observation for signs of hemorrhage important in the postoperative nursing care of the amputee?

Because major blood vessels are severed during the surgical procedure.

18 The nurse has noted that the amputee's pulse is rapid and thready and that his blood pressure is 15 points lower than the previous reading. What should the nurse do?

a. Elevate the foot of the bed.
b. Look under the stump to check amount of blood loss.
c. If necessary, apply pressure or the tourniquet.
d. Call the physician.

a. _____
b. _____
c. _____
d. _____

19 Postoperatively, pain is generally not intense for either an upper or lower extremity amputee since the incision is not usually over a movable joint. Therefore, when pain is intense, complications are highly possible and the patient should be observed closely. The nurse checks the amputee closely for indications of _____ and _____ .

hemorrhage

pain

20 A prosthesis is often essential to the patient's regaining the function of the affected extremity. Prevention of complications that would preclude use of a prosthesis thus becomes one of the goals of the amputee's postoperative nursing care. One complication to be prevented is the development of extreme adduction or abduction, flexion, and external rotation contractures. List three basic goals of the amputee's postoperative nursing care plan.

a. To assist the patient in the grieving process.

a. _____
_____

b. To assist the patient to regain function.
c. To prevent complications such as contractures. *(Review Chapter 2 if you have forgotten what a contracture is.)*

b. _____
_____
c. _____
_____

21 After amputation of the lower limb, the amputee's stump should be positioned to prevent flexion contractures. The patient should be instructed not to place a pillow under his stump (or under his knee if the amputation has been below the knee). Postoperative nursing care of the lower limb amputee should be focused on the prevention of contractures; the types are _____,

adduction

abduction; flexion

external rotation

_____, _____, and _____.

22 If the patient is permitted to remain sitting in a chair for a long time, hip and/or knee flexion contractures will result. The patient should change his position frequently and should lie on his abdomen for 30 minutes three or four times per day. Which part of Fig. 13-5 demonstrates the correct way to position the patient after an amputation? Why?

B; In order to prevent contractures, the limb should be extended.

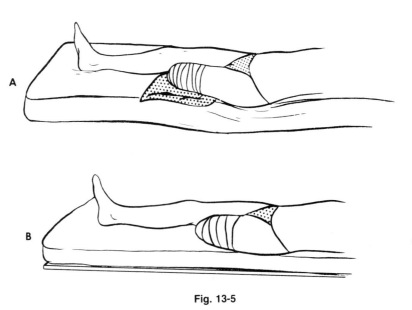

Fig. 13-5

23 List three instructions to be given to the lower limb amputee regarding the prevention of contractures.

a. No pillows are to be placed under the stump.

a. _____
_____

b. Position should be changed frequently.
c. Lie on abdomen for 30 minutes 3 or 4 times per day.

b. _____
   _____
   _____

c. _____
   _____

24 The patient may continue to experience tingling, itching, or other sensations in the amputated portion of the extremity for some time after surgery. However, these *phantom sensations* tend to decrease with the resumption of extremity activity. Postoperatively, the

phantom sensations

amputee may experience _____ .

25 Eight to ten days after surgery, the amputee may experience pain in the amputated portion of the extremity. The patient should be told to expect phantom pain and that, like the phantom sensations, it will diminish over time. Phantom sensation and phantom pain

are not

(are? are not?) the same.

26 Phantom limb pain tends to occur when the patient has had preoperative pain in the limb and when he has trigger zones which produce painful spasm in phantom limb when stimulated. Phantom limb pain may be relieved by the application of pressure to the stump or ambulation with a prosthesis. Similarly, phantom sensations may be relieved by stump muscular activity. Three days after a right below-the-knee amputation, the patient complains that his right foot

That he is having phantom sensations, which may last for some time but they will "improve" as he walks more.

itches. What would the nurse tell him?

27 Resumption of normal function after an amputation of the lower extremity includes walking and weight-bearing. At the time of surgery, the orthopedic surgeon may apply a plaster cast to the lower limb. The cast is held in place by a system of shoulder straps similar to common suspenders or is attached to a waist band. A metal socket at the distal end of the cast permits attachment of a pylon for ambulation, as shown in Fig. 13-6. The use of a pylon permits early

ambulation; weight-bearing

_____ and _____ .

28 The plaster cast maintains the position of the extremity so contractures are prevented; prevents the development of postoperative stump edema, which leads to better stump shaping; decreases pain; and aids hemostasis. However, as with any plaster cast, the wound is covered and pressure necrosis is a possible complication. List the advantages of the use of a plaster cast and pylon attachment on a lower limb amputation.

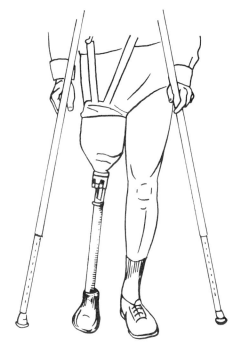

Fig. 13-6. Anterior view of plaster cast with pylon attachment, after above-the-knee amputation.

a. Permits early ambulation and weight-bearing
b. Prevents contractures
c. Prevents postoperative edema
d. Decreases pain
e. Aids hemostasis

a. _____
b. _____
c. _____
d. _____
e. _____

29 The shoulder straps should be checked periodically to see that they are adequately supporting the cast. It is possible that the cast may fall off soon after surgery because of changes in the size of the stump. If this does occur, the nurse may apply a pressure dressing with a cotton elastic bandage until the cast can be reapplied. If signs of loosening are present, the cast may be changed 2 weeks after surgery. If the cast comes off or is removed, the stump should be checked for _____ and _____
_____ .

wound healing; pressure necrosis

30 Amputation of the upper extremity frequently results from traumatic injury and there is little time for appropriate psychological preparation. The traumatic upper extremity amputee's psychological adaptation is not predictable because it is not known where the amputee will start in the grief process. Those around the amputee such as family and friends will influence the patient's adjustment. Grieving over the loss of all or part of an extremity is (abnormal? normal?).

normal

214

31 Since there currently is no immediate postoperative cast and prosthesis system for the upper extremity, the patient's rehabilitation is delayed until the stump is healed and shaped. The inability to use the extremity contributes to the patient's difficulty in adapting to the loss. Prosthesis fitting depends on there being a _____ and _____ stump.

32 In order to be able to use a prosthesis on either an upper or a lower extremity, the patient must have a well-healed, well-shaped stump with the stump skin in good condition. The basic element of stump care is skin care. The nurse is responsible for teaching and supervising stump skin care.

33 The patient should actively participate in caring for his stump while in the hospital since he should be becoming independent. Each day, after the sutures are removed, the patient should wash the stump with soap and warm water, rinse it well, and dry it thoroughly. The patient begins caring for his stump _____ _____ .

34 Unless prescribed by the physician, oil, alcohol, and powders should not be used on the stump since they may soften or dry the skin excessively. After the stump is bathed, it should be exposed to the air for approximately 20 minutes. List the steps of daily stump care.

a. _____
b. _____
c. _____
d. _____

35 As the amputee cares for his stump, he should examine it for signs of complications. He should be taught to watch for swelling, calluses, rash or blisters, and changes in the color or appearance of the skin. The amputee may be unable to use a prothesis if any or all of the following complications are present: changes in skin color or _____ , rash or _____ , _____ , _____ , or _____ .

36 The skin on the stump must be in condition to withstand the pressure of the prosthesis socket. Signs of skin breakdown include _____ , _____ _____ , and _____ _____ .

37 In addition to the prevention of contractures, proper positioning of the patient is important to prevent stump edema that would also preclude use of a prosthesis. Why is each of the positions shown in Fig. 13-7 incorrect?

a. Could form flexion contracture

b. Could form adduction contracture

c. Could form flexion contracture and could develop stump edema

a. _____

b. _____

c. _____

Fig. 13-7

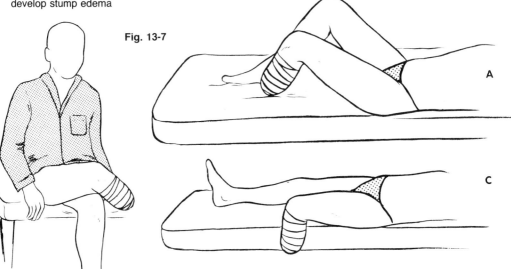

B

38 Not all amputations result in a closed, well-formed stump because of the nature of the surgical procedure and the reason for the amputation. The physician may prescribe bandaging the patient's stump to reduce the stump edema or to mold it for prosthesis fitting. The patient should be encouraged to prepare for ambulation and a prosthesis because it will assist him to return to normal functioning and decrease the _____.

phantom sensations

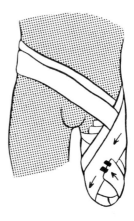

Fig. 13-8. A shrinker bandage is applied to the stump to reduce stump edema and to mold the stump.

39 If the stump wound is left open to drain, extension traction may be applied to hold the skin flaps so that they do not retract, leaving the end of the bone exposed. The types of amputations that may be performed are _____ , _____ , _____ .

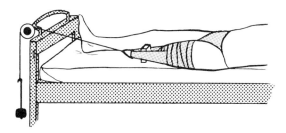

Fig. 13-9. Extension traction on the stump after amputation.

40 A prosthesis must be fitted and adjusted by a person trained in the technique. In most institutions this is done in the physical therapy department, which also trains the amputee how to use the prosthesis. The nurse is responsible for assisting and supervising the amputee in the care of his stump and prosthesis. In order to care for himself and his stump, the amputee needs to know:

a. How to prevent contractures
b. The steps of the amputation procedure
c. The signs of complications
d. How to wash his stump

41 The socket of the prosthesis must be kept clean. Since both the stump and the socket must be thoroughly dried, the best time to clean them is at night. With slight modification, the socket is cleansed in the same manner as the stump. The steps of stump hygiene are _____

_____ , _____ , and _____ .

42 Although the physical therapist teaches the amputee how to function with his prosthesis, the nurse must be familiar with the training program in order to assist and encourage the patient. Unlike the stump, the prosthesis socket cannot be immersed in water but must be wiped out with a damp cloth. The nurse's responsibilities in the care of the amputee are:

a. Teaching the patient to care for his stump
b. Teaching the patient to use a prosthesis
c. Supervising the patient as he cares for his stump
d. Encouraging the patient in the use of his prosthesis
e. Fitting the prosthesis

43 The amputee must maintain full use of the other extremities during his hospitalization to enable him to resume normal activities. Often the lower limb amputee must use crutches while the prosthesis is being fitted and while he is learning to use it. Use of a trapeze, weight-lifting, exercises, and a program of physical therapy are helpful in maintaining and improving the status of the other extremities. Exercises of the limb stump are also beneficial because ____

they help prevent contractures and decrease phantom sensation

_____
_____ .

44 If the amputee has a contracture of the knee above the stump, he (can? cannot?) use a prosthesis.

cannot

45 The measures that can be used to maintain the function of the amputee's other extremities are (weight-lifting? active exercises? use of a trapeze? traction and splints?).

weight-lifting, active exercises, use of a trapeze

46 The physician may prescribe stump bandaging (to protect the skin? to reduce edema? to mold the stump?).

to reduce edema, to mold the stump

47 Stump traction may be necessary:
a. If the stump wound is infected
b. If the stump wound is healing too slowly
c. If the stump wound is left open to drain
d. If the patient is developing contractures

c

48 The purpose of stump traction is to _____

hold the skin flaps so that they will not retract, leaving the end of the bone exposed

_____
_____ .

49 Itching, tingling, or other feelings in the part of the extremity that was removed are _____ .

phantom sensations

50 Phantom sensations are treated by:
a. Removal of the nerves in the stump
b. Weight-bearing on the stump
c. Injections of local anesthetics in the stump
d. Ambulation
e. Increasing extremity activity

b, d, and e

51 The amputee must be taught to check his stump for _____

rashes or blisters; swelling; changes in skin color or appearance

_____ , _____ , and
_____ .

52 The amputee must also know how to care for his _____

stump

prosthesis

and _____ .

53 Before the amputation is performed, nursing care of the patient

psychological preparation is focused on _____ .

54 In the immediate postoperative phase, nursing care is focused
on:

b and d
a. Preventing contractures
b. Observing the patient for signs of shock
c. Teaching the patient to care for his stump
d. Observing the patient for signs of hemorrhage

55 Mr. Jones has just had his left leg amputated 1 inch above the
knee. The nurse is watching him closely for signs of hemorrhage
because:

b
a. Amputees bleed more easily than other patients
b. Major blood vessels were severed and sutured during the procedure
c. Infection could cause necrosis of a blood vessel

56 The nurse has taken Mr. Jones' pulse and blood pressure; the

the stump dressing, under
his stump for drainage
nurse should also check (his temperature? the stump dressing? under
his stump for drainage? for phantom sensations?).

57 The nurse would report to the physician if Mr. Jones' pulse is

rapid or thready _____ ; if his blood pressure is

lower; saturated _____ than before; or if his dressing is _____ .
If Mr. Jones is hemorrhaging, the nurse would elevate (the head

the foot of the bed of the bed? his stump on a pillow? the foot of the bed?).

58 Contractures can be prevented by having Mr. Jones:

b and c
a. Sit in a chair most of the time
b. Lie prone several times a day
c. Keep his stump flat when in bed

59 The nurse should instruct Mr. Jones to use (alcohol? mineral

soap and water oil? soap and water? lanolin? talcum powder?) on his stump.

60 Several days after surgery, Mr. Jones' stump is edematous. To

shrinker bandage reduce the swelling, the nurse could apply a(n) _____

_____ .

61 Mr. Jones will be trained to use his prosthesis by the (physician?

physical therapist physical therapist? nurse?).

62 After Mr. Jones is fitted for a prosthesis, the nurse is responsible
for:

All of these
a. Supervising him as he uses it
b. Teaching him to care for it
c. Supervising him as he cares for his stump
d. Encouraging him as he uses the prosthesis

63 The main goal of Mr. Jones' nursing care plan was:

b

a. To restore the affected part
b. To assist him to return to normal activity
c. To teach him to live within his limitations

PRINCIPLES OF NURSING CARE OF THE NONSURGICAL ORTHOPEDIC PATIENT

Patients with metabolic disorders, minor traumatic injuries, and inflammatory diseases are most often cared for by the nurse in the physician's office, outpatient department, or neighborhood health center, and by the visiting nurse. The hospital nurse has contact with these patients only when they are acutely ill or are hospitalized for corrective therapy. Therefore, the primary nursing care goal for these patients is to prepare them to care for themselves at home. This goal necessitates helping the patient to understand and accept his diagnosis and treatment, assisting him to function independently within his limitations, and teaching him and his family how to perform selected procedures.

CHAPTER 14

Principles of nursing care of the patient with a metabolic disorder

■ Just as red blood cells are continuously being produced and destroyed by the body, bone tissue also is in a state of constant flux. The metabolic disorders are so named because they are associated with disturbances in the production and destruction of bone cells, and they are related either to the dietary intake of an appropriate nutrient or the bone cells' supply, storage, or utilization of one or more specific nutrients. One advantage of our affluent society is that there has been a decrease in the number of patients with bone deformities and metabolic bone disorders related to malnutrition. Rickets, scurvy, and osteomalacia are metabolic disorders that have become uncommon in American society. Since these disorders are encountered infrequently, the nurse caring for such patients should seek pertinent information regarding their nursing care from other relevant literature sources. Rather than dealing with the metabolic disorders in a comprehensive manner, this chapter focuses on the two most common metabolic disorders—osteoporosis and gout.

b

1 Osteoporosis is a process of gradual loss of the bone in which the bones become porous and brittle; that is, there is a diffuse reduction in bone density that results when the rate of bone resorption exceeds the rate of bone formation. Osteoporosis can best be described as:
a. A chemical imbalance
b. A change in the normal pattern of bone flux
c. A nutritional disease
d. Bone malnutrition

porous

2 When the patient has osteoporosis, a roentgenogram will show that the involved bones are _____.

estrogen levels

steroid therapy; immobilization

3 The normal cycle of bone formation and resorption may be interrupted by a number of factors. Decreased estrogen levels, immobilization, steroid therapy, and idiopathic causes are thought to be factors in the development of osteoporosis. Three specific causative factors in osteoporosis are _____,
_____, and _____.

223

4 Osteoporosis is most frequently seen in postmenopausal women because of the relationship between estrogen production and bone anabolism. Anabolism refers to the process of tissue or bone

formation _____ , while catabolism refers to the pro-

destruction cess of tissue or bone _____ .

5 Osteoporosis in an older woman may first be evidenced by the development of a ''dowager's hump'' (dorsal kyphosis) or severe low back pain. Other patients may be diagnosed only after incurring a fracture as a result of minor trauma. Which of the following may be indicative of osteoporosis?

c and d a. Dorsal scoliosis

b. Steroid therapy over an extended period of time

c. Severe low back pain

d. Fractured hip resulting from sitting forcefully

6 Other bones besides the vertebrae may be sites of osteoporosis. These other sites are the pelvis, hands, wrists, and the femoral neck. These additional osteoporotic sites may similarly show evidence of

reduction in bone density _____

porous by appearing _____ on x-ray.

7 In a previous frame it was noted that some cases of osteoporosis are diagnosed only after the patient has sustained a fracture as a result of minor trauma. This phenomenon occurs because osteo-

brittle porotic bones are _____ .

8 The preceding statements suggest a nursing care goal: to prevent

fractures _____ .

9 Drug therapy in the treatment of osteoporosis is usually limited to the administration of estrogens. However, intravenous adminis-tration of calcium, calcitonin, and/or fluoride may be prescribed. Estrogens may be recommended either to prevent or to treat osteo-porosis in postmenopausal women. Osteoporotic patients are treated

fluoride, estrogens, calcitonin with (fluoride? estrogens? phosphates? calcitonin? steroids?).

10 In addition, the dietary intake of calcium and protein must be adequate regardless of the causative factors associated with osteo-porosis. Nursing care of the osteoporotic patient is focused on the

fractures prevention of _____ and on the patient's

nutrition _____ .

11 Hormonal therapy generates implications for nursing actions that are related to the type of therapy rather than to the condition being treated. It is the nurse's responsibility to be aware of these implications in order to provide the appropriate nursing care. Which of the following nursing actions would be appropriate in caring for a post-menopausal patient on estrogen therapy?

All of these

a. Assess patient's posture at time therapy is initiated
b. Teach patient about home hazards that may cause her to fall
c. Remind patient of need for annual cancer check-up
d. Encourage patient to be physically active

12 Senile and chronically ill patients develop disuse osteoporosis since the bone matrix is not stimulated. Mr. Jones sustained multiple fractures and has been in traction for 4 weeks. The nurse is concerned that he may develop osteoporosis since one of the factors

immobilization

associated with its development is _____.

13 The therapy employed in the prevention and treatment of osteoporosis caused by immobilization is to increase the amount of activity through active and/or passive exercise, since activity stimu-

can

lates the bone matrix. Osteoporosis caused by immobilization (can? cannot?) be prevented.

14 Because of the limitations on movement imposed by his being in traction, Mr. Jones may be unable to actively exercise. Therefore, the nurse must identify joint motions that are permissible and develop an exercise program within the framework of his limitations. Which of the following nursing care elements are important in the prevention and treatment of osteoporosis?

a, b, and d

a   Prevention of fractures
b. Patient education regarding medications
c. Dietary intake of carbohydrates
d. Patient activity regimen

15 *Gout* is considered to be a metabolic disorder because it is the result of underexcretion, overproduction, or a combination of underexcretion and overproduction of uric acid. The excess uric acid accumulates as deposits of urate salt crystals. In gout, uric acid is

excessively; minimally

produced (minimally? excessively?) and/or excreted (minimally? excessively?).

16 The Arthritis Foundation classifies gout as a form of arthritis since the urate salt crystals tend to be deposited in and around joints. However, the urate salt crystals may also be deposited on periarticular and subcutaneous tissue or in the kidneys. These deposits are seen most often in the soft tissue of the ear, the olecranon bursa, and patellar bursa. Gout may be considered as a metabolic disease be-

overproduced

cause uric acid may be (underproduced? overproduced?).

225

17 The deposits of urate salts, referred to as *tophi,* can cause damage to and destruction of the joints. Which statement is true?

b

a. Tophi are deposits of uric acid.

b. Tophi are deposits of urate salts.

18 The early phase of gout, hyperuricemia, is asymptomatic, but as the tophi enlarge the patient experiences intense pain in the involved joint(s). The involved joints, usually in the toes, become red, edematous, tender, and limited in motion. Gout may be evidenced by:

a, b, c, and e

a. A reddened, painful toe joint

b. An edematous toe joint

c. An elevated serum uric acid level

d. Red, swollen feet

e. A painfully tender toe joint

f. Metabolic disorders

19 The clinical course of gout is characterized by periods of remission and exacerbation; that is, gout is a chronic condition. Over time, the deposits of urate crystals may lead to some crippling or deformity, and eventually renal complications may occur, especially if the gout remains untreated. Indicate which statements are true.

a, b, d, and f

a. Gout is indirectly caused by a metabolic disorder.

b. Gout is a form of arthritis.

c. Uric acid is deposited in a joint in gout.

d. Gout is a chronic disease.

e. The gout patient always has pain.

f. Gout may be associated with foot deformities.

20 During the acute phase of gout, medical treatment and nursing care are concentrated on alleviation of the patient's pain. The patient is placed on bedrest, and a bed cradle or other device is placed over the patient's feet to prevent contact with bed linens. Use of a bed cradle is consistent with the nursing care objective of _____

alleviating pain

_____ .

21 Nursing measures such as applications of ice or moist heat may also be instrumental in alleviating the patient's pain. The gout patient experiences pain during a(n) (remission? exacerbation?).

exacerbation

22 The physician most frequently prescribes colchicine for an acute attack of gout. However, the colchicine dosage must be individually adjusted because of its toxic side effects. It is given as prescribed until the patient's pain is less severe or until the patient experiences abdominal cramping, diarrhea, nausea, or vomiting. An acute attack of gout may be treated by administering, as prescribed, _____ .

colchicine

abdominal cramping; nausea;
diarrhea; vomiting

23 Mr. Brown has been admitted to the hospital for treatment of gout. The physician has prescribed colchicine. Four toxic side effects that might result from the medication are _____

_____ , _____ , _____ ,

and _____ .

pain

24 Colchicine may be administered intravenously but the parenteral route eliminates the gastrointestinal signs of toxicity. However, the nurse will be able to observe any reduction in _____ .

25 Phenylbutazone, indomethacin, or corticotropin may be prescribed during an acute exacerbation of gout if the drug of choice produces toxic side effects. The drug of choice in the acute phase is

colchicine

_____ .

26 The nurse makes the patient with gouty toe joints more comfortable by _____ ,

putting him in bed; placing a
bed cradle over his feet;
applying moist heat or ice to
his feet; giving him the prescribed medications
(any three, any order)

_____ , and _____

_____ .

27 Phenylbutazone, indomethacin, or corticotropin may be administered to aid uric acid clearance and because of their anti-inflammatory properties. These drugs are administered during the (chronic? acute?) phase.

acute

28 After the acute phase has been controlled, uricosuric therapy is used to prevent the development of tophi or to resolve existing tophi. The term uricosuric implies that medications are given to:

c

a. Stop production of uric acid
b. Decrease production of uric acid
c. Increase excretion of uric acid
d. Stop excretion or uric acid

29 Uricosuric agents present implications for nursing care, since the patient must understand that he must take the drug for the remainder of his life to prevent the development of tophi and the accompanying renal complications. Uricosuric agents include probenecid (Benemid), sulfinpyrazone (Anturane), zoxazolamine (Flexin), and large doses (more than 3 Gm. per day) or acetylsalicylic acid. Match the medications with the appropriate phrase.

c, e
a, b, d
a, b, d
e

_____ 1. Colchicine   a. Long-range therapy
_____ 2. Sulfinpyrazone   b. Prevent development of tophi
_____ 3. Probenecid   c. Toxic side effects
_____ 4. Phenylbutazone   d. Increase uric acid excretion
                                       e. Acute phase

30 Until the dosage of the uricosuric agent has been adjusted, the patient must be observed for indications of an acute attack, since the medication may cause the urates to be mobilized too quickly. The physician may prescribe allopurinol as long-range therapy to prevent the overproduction of uric acid. Allopurinol may be given in combination with probenecid or other _____ agents.

uricosuric

31 Administration of these drugs requires that the patient's urine volume be maintained at adequate levels. List four nursing care orders that would be appropriate for a gout patient.

a. Force fluids
b. Instruct patient regarding importance of continued therapy
c. Observe patient for signs of acute attack
d. Measure urinary output

a. _____

b. _____

c. _____

d. _____

prevent
overproduction

32 Allopurinol is administered to (increase? prevent? decrease?) (excretion? underproduction? overproduction?) of uric acid.

33 In the past, gout was associated with ingestion of large amounts of purine-containing foods, which were associated with dietary indiscretion. Dietary restriction of purine intake formerly was the mainstay of therapy. Today, the physician may or may not advise the patient to restrict his purine intake. If purines are restricted, the nurse must be prepared to assist the patient in understanding the rationale for doing so. The drugs described in the preceding frames are prescribed to control the metabolic disorder that results in tophi formation. The metabolic disorder is characterized by

underexcretion; overproduction; a combination of both underexcretion and overproduction

_____ , _____ ,

or _____

_____ of uric acid.

34 Which of the following are metabolic disorders?

a, b, and d

a. Scurvy   c. Arthritis
b. Osteoporosis   d. Gout

porous
brittle

35 Osteoporotic bones can be described as being _____ and _____ .

36 The anatomic structures most affected by gout are the

joints

_____ .

37 Indicate whether each of the following medications is (1) used in the treatment or prevention of gout, (2) used in the treatment or prevention of osteoporosis, or (3) not used in either of these conditions:

1	2
3	1
2	1
1	1
2	1

(Small doses of aspirin inhibit excretion of uric acid; large doses have uricosuric effect.)

_____ Allopurinol   _____ Fluoride

_____ Aspirin (small doses)   _____ Indomethacin

_____ Calcitonin   _____ Phenylbutazone

_____ Colchicine   _____ Sulfinpyrazone

_____ Estrogen   _____ Steroids

38 List four nursing care objectives for a postmenopausal osteoporosis patient.

a. Prevent fractures
b. Increase activity
c. Improve calcium and protein intake
d. Instruct patient regarding estrogen therapy

a. _____

b. _____

c. _____

d. _____

39 Which of the following nursing observations and measurements should be performed when the patient has gout?

a and d
(b and c are appropriate for osteoporotic patient.)

a. Measure urinary output
b. Observe posture before treatment is initiated
c. Observe that dietary intake of calcium is adequate
d. Observe for indications of nausea
e. Observe for indications of nerve damage in feet

40 Mr. White is to be discharged from the hospital in the near future. The physician has indicated that Mr. White will be on uricosuric therapy. The nurse has talked with Mr. White and has found that he does not plan to take his medication after he gets home. The nurse realizes that it is essential that he do so in order to _____

resolve existing tophi; prevent further development of tophi

_____ and to

_____

_____ .

41 The development of tophi must be prevented since they may

renal; orthopedic
(e.g., deformities)

generate _____ and _____ complications.

42 Briefly describe why nutrition is a relevant topic in orthopedic nursing.

Reread the introduction to this chapter. *(If you question the correctness of your response, discuss it with your instructor.)*

CHAPTER 15

Principles of nursing care of the patient with traumatic injuries

■ As has been mentioned in previous chapters, much of the orthopedic surgeon's time is spent caring for the patient who has been injured in an accident. Many of these patients are cared for in the physician's office or the emergency room of the hospital. Since fractures have already been discussed, they will be omitted from this chapter, although they are among the common traumatic injuries. The nursing care of patients with traumatic injuries focuses on relieving the symptoms and teaching the patient to care for himself at home so that he will eventually be able to resume normal functions.

<table>
<tr><td>fractures
sprains; strains
contusions</td><td>**1** Many kinds of trauma result in injury to the musculoskeletal system. Some frequently occurring injuries to the soft tissues of the musculoskeletal system are *sprains, strains,* and *contusions.* Injuries to the bones are _____, while injuries to the soft tissues are _____, _____, and _____ .</td></tr>
<tr><td>joint</td><td>**2** There is no consensus among physicians regarding definition of the terms strain and sprain. However, an injury to the ligaments around a joint is usually labeled a *sprain.* Sprains may be of varying degrees of severity. The involved ligament(s) may be stretched, torn slightly, or completely severed. Sprains are injuries to the ligaments supporting a _____ .</td></tr>
<tr><td>stretched
torn</td><td>**3** Severe sprains may also disrupt the joint's synovial lining, which may be followed by hemorrhage into the joint. A sprain may be minor—the involved ligaments are _____ ; or it may be more severe—the involved ligaments are _____ .</td></tr>
<tr><td>ligaments
muscles</td><td>**4** An injury to the muscles is usually labeled a *strain.* Sprains are injuries to _____, while strains involve _____ .</td></tr>
<tr><td></td><td>**5** In both sprains and strains the injury results from an excessive or forceful pull (stretch) being exerted on the involved area. When a</td></tr>
</table>

sprain occurs, the affected area or joint becomes painful and swollen.

pain; edema

Two symptoms of sprains are _____ and _____ .

6 A strain tears muscle fibers during forceful use. Usually the patient is able to identify a specific, severe, disabling onset of the pain. When a runner complains of having "pulled" a muscle and can

strained

no longer run, he probably has _____ the muscle.

7 Selection of first-aid measures, medical treatment, and nursing care is based on knowledge of the processes occurring as a result of injury. The emphasis of nursing care for the patient with a sprain or strain is on patient teaching; the nurse must teach the patient how to care for himself at home.

8 The edema that may occur after a sprain or strain is caused by concomitant tearing of small blood vessels, which results in interstitial hemorrhage and interruption of lymphatic drainage. The presence of edema suggests that the affected extremity should be

elevated

_____ .

9 Elevation of the affected extremity will help to prevent or to reduce edema while simultaneously permitting the affected part to rest and heal. Applications of ice during the first 24 hours after injury prevent or reduce edema as well as control hemorrhage and ease pain. Therefore, the nurse should teach the patient how to perform which of the following actions:

b and d
(The entire extremity must be elevated to be effective.)

a. Application of adhesive splints
b. Application of ice bags
c. Elevation of the affected part
d. Elevation of the affected extremity

10 The pain, tenderness, or muscle spasms associated with sprains result from stimulation of the nerve endings. When soft tissues are

torn

injured, small blood vessels are _____, lymphatic drainage is

interrupted; stimulated

_____ , and nerve endings are _____ .

11 Since the ligaments have been torn or severed to some degree in a sprain, they must be immobilized to permit healing. The physician may immobilize the affected joint by splinting it with layers of adhesive tape or specialized bandaging. (Occasionally, the physician may apply a cast.) A splint is applied to the affected joint to

immobilize

_____ it.

12 A Shanz or Robert Jones' bandage may be used to immobilize the affected area after a sprain or strain is incurred. A Shanz dressing is comprised of alternate layers of sheet wadding (as is used for

231

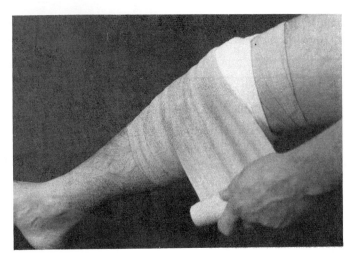

Fig. 15-1. Shanz dressing, consisting of alternate layers of sheet wadding and ace bandages, is applied from ankle to mid-thigh.

padding under a cast) and Ace bandages. The Shanz dressing, used most frequently for knee sprains, extends from the ankle to mid-thigh. A Shanz dressing applied from ankle to mid-thigh will

immobilize a sprained knee _____ .

13 A Robert Jones' bandage is comprised of alternate layers of bulky cotton and Ace bandages. Both dressings are applied with some pressure by stretching the elastic bandage as it is unrolled to create a compression force. This pressure helps to reduce and/or

edema prevent _____ .

14 To summarize, the basic elements of treatment of the patient with a sprain or strain are immobilization and elevation of the affected extremity and the application of pressure and ice. Match the elements of treatment with the appropriate rationale.

c   _____ 1. Immobilization of affected joint

a, d   _____ 2. Elevation of the affected extremity

a, b, d   _____ 3. Application of pressure to affected area

a, b, d   _____ 4. Application of ice to affected area

a. To reduce edema
b. To control hemorrhage
c. To permit healing
d. To prevent edema

15 A *dislocation* occurs when the ligaments supporting a joint tear, permitting displacement of the joint surfaces. The hip, knee, elbow, and shoulder are the joints most often dislocated. The signs and symptoms of a dislocated joint are pain, immobility, and deformity. Indicate whether the following statements are true or false.

232

_____ a. A dislocation is caused by torn ligaments and slipping joints.

_____ b. A dislocation results from torn ligaments, which allow the joint surfaces to slip out of place.

16 Dislocations are treated by returning the joint surfaces to their normal articulations and immobilizing the joint while healing occurs. A dislocation should be reduced as soon as possible because damage to the muscles, blood vessels, nerves, and tendons around a dislocated joint increase in direct proportion to the length of time the reduction is delayed. Match the signs and symptoms with the appropriate injury.

_____ 1. Sprains   a. Immobility
_____ 2. Dislocation b. Pain
                        c. Edema
                        d. Deformity

17 Reduction of a dislocation is the process of returning the joint surfaces to their normal articulations. Match the type of reduction with the appropriate phrase.

_____ 1. Open reduction   a. Realignment of the fragments
_____ 2. Closed reduction   while the patient is sedated
                             b. Surgical intervention to realign
                                the fragments

18 Closed reduction is the preferred method of treating a dislocation. Closed reduction of a dislocation could then be defined as:

a. The use of a surgical procedure to return the joints to their articulations
b. The process of returning the joint surfaces to their articulations while the patient is sedated or anesthetized
c. The process of returning the joint fragments to their normal alignment while the patient is sedated

19 An open reduction is utilized to treat a dislocation if the position of the torn ligaments precludes closed reduction. The factor that

makes an open reduction necessary is the _____

_____ .

20 Some patients are able to reduce their dislocation without assistance. The associated hazard is that the end of the torn ligament may be interposed between the joint surfaces. Necrosis of the end of the ligament may result from the articulating joint surface's pressure.

Location of the ligament (can? cannot?) be determined radiologically.

21 Some patients repeatedly dislocate the same joint, in which case metallic fixation or surgical repair of the tendons or transfer of muscles may be employed at the time of open reduction to prevent future dislocation of the joint. A joint that has been dislocated for the first time is treated by:

b

a. Immobilization in a plaster cast
b. Closed reduction when possible
c. Open reduction and metallic fixation

22 When possible, a dislocation of the shoulder joint is treated by closed reduction. After reduction, the affected arm is immobilized, permitting the joint to rest and heal. The signs and symptoms

discomfort, loss of motion,
deformed appearance

of a dislocation are (discomfort? loss of motion? swelling? deformed appearance?).

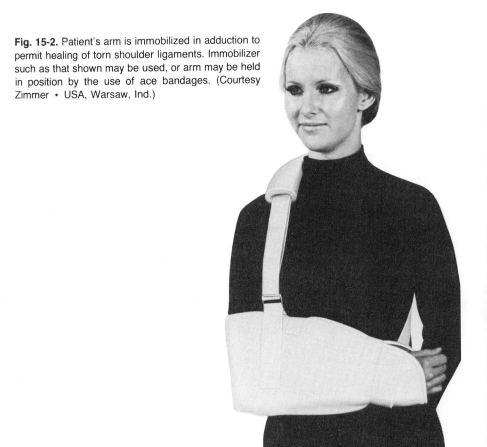

Fig. 15-2. Patient's arm is immobilized in adduction to permit healing of torn shoulder ligaments. Immobilizer such as that shown may be used, or arm may be held in position by the use of ace bandages. (Courtesy Zimmer • USA, Warsaw, Ind.)

23 After the ligaments around the shoulder joint have healed, the immobilizer is removed and exercises are begun to strengthen

the ligaments. The affected arm was immobilized to permit the
joint _____ to _____ and _____ .

ligaments; rest; heal

24 A sprain of either or both collateral ligaments of the knee is
caused by forceful abduction of the extended knee. A bruise, edema,
and tenderness are symptoms of a collateral ligament sprain. Knee
sprains are treated in much the same way as other sprains. List the
four basic elements of treatment for sprains and strains.

a. _____

b. _____

c. _____

d. _____

a. Immobilization of affected
joint
b. Elevation of the affected
extremity
c. Application of pressure to
the affected area
d. Application of ice to the
affected area

25 A sprained knee can be immobilized by applying a _____
or _____ bandage.

Shanz
Robert Jones'

26 As the sprained knee heals, the patient should begin doing
quadriceps setting exercises. After an injury, exercises are done to:
a. Prevent future injuries
b. Promote healing
c. Strengthen the affected ligaments
d. Realign the joint surfaces

a and c

27 Since the patient with a strain or a sprain must know how to
care for himself at home, the nurse should teach him:
a. Not to do exercises after the extremity heals
b. Not to remove the adhesive tape, Shanz, or Robert Jones' bandage until the physician tells him to
c. How to elevate the affected extremity
d. How to apply moist heat

b and c

28 A strained or sprained ankle can be immobilized by:
a. Applying a plaster cast
b. Surrounding it with icebags
c. Splinting it with adhesive tape
d. Doing a closed reduction

a and c

29 In a dislocation, the joint surfaces are:
a. Torn out of place
b. Displaced when the ligaments tear
c. Not in their normal articulations
d. Injured by forceful abduction

b and c

30 Quadriceps setting exercises are used to strengthen the knee

collateral ligaments   after a sprain of the _____
                        has healed.

31 Match the signs and symptoms with the appropriate injury.

a, d   _____ 1. Sprained ankle   a. Pain
a, b, c   _____ 2. Dislocated elbow   b. Stiffness
                                            c. Deformity
                                            d. Edema

32 Match the methods of treatment with the appropriate injury.

d, e, f   _____ 1. Sprained knee   a. Open reduction
b, d, e   _____ 2. Sprained wrist   b. Splint with tape
a, c, e   _____ 3. Dislocated shoulder c. Closed reduction
                                            d. Apply icebags
                                            e. Immobilization
                                            f. Apply Shanz dressing

33 Nursing care of the patient centers on:

b   a. Splinting the injured part
              b. Teaching the patient how to care for himself
              c. Teaching the patient to apply splints

elevating the affected   **34** The sprain patient must be taught to prevent edema by _____
extremity; applying   _____
icebags   and _____ .

35 In addition to knowledge of operative orthopedics, the nurse in
the physician's office or hospital emergency room should also know:

All of these   a. Basic first aid techniques
                b. What community resources are available to the patient who will
                   be caring for himself at home
                c. How to be an effective teacher
                d. How to use and teach good body mechanics

CHAPTER 16

Principles of nursing care of the patient with an inflammatory condition

■ Current research in arthritis suggests that many inflammatory conditions and diseases are variant forms of arthritis and should be classified as rheumatic diseases. Since it would be impractical to study all types of rheumatic diseases, two common types of arthritis that are meaningful for orthopedic nurses have been selected for intensive study in this chapter. Also included in this chapter are osteomyelitis and inflammatory conditions that tend to be related to specific anatomic structures.

inflammatory condition

1 *Tenosynovitis* is an inflammation of the synovial sheath that covers a tendon. Tenosynovitis is a(n) (metabolic disorder? congenital disease? inflammatory condition?).

d

2 A strain of or a traumatic injury to the tendon is often associated with tenosynovitis, which is characterized by the presence of localized swelling and tenderness. In tenosynovitis:
a. The tendon is infected
b. The synovial sheath is infected
c. The synovial sheath is inflamed
d. The synovial sheath of a tendon is inflamed

tenderness
swelling

3 The affected area is treated by immobilization and applications of heat. Two signs of tenosynovitis are _____ and _____ of the area.

hot compresses (as a source of heat), a plaster cast (as a means of immobilizing the part)

4 As with most other orthopedic disorders, the affected extremity or part is immobilized in a functional position. The treatment of tenosynovitis also includes the application of (cold compresses? hot compresses? an icebag? a plaster cast?).

prevent the spread of infection

5 If the tenosynovitis is localized with the formation of an abscess, the physician often elects to open and drain the abscess to prevent spread of the infection. The physician incises and drains the area affected by tenosynovitis to (relieve the pain? reduce the edema? speed healing? prevent the spread of infection?).

237

6 If the patient has tenosynovitis of the fingers, the physician may place a splint on the patient's hand to immobilize them. The fingers would be positioned so they are (extended? spread apart? slightly flexed? in a fist?).

slightly flexed
(functional position)

7 *Synovitis* is an inflammation of the synovial membrane with which a joint capsule is lined. When the synovial sheath of a tendon is inflamed, the diagnosis is _____. When the synovial membrane of a joint capsule is inflamed, the diagnosis is _____.

tenosynovitis

synovitis

8 *Chondritis* is inflammation of a cartilage; *myositis* is inflammation of a muscle. Inflammatory conditions of the musculoskeletal system include:

b, c, d, and e
a. Cellulitis
b. Chondritis
c. Synovitis
d. Myositis
e. Tenosynovitis
f. Rhinitis

9 The nursing care of the patient with either synovitis, chondritis, or myositis is concentrated on the relief of discomfort and the prevention of deformities. The affected part is maintained in normal alignment and is immobilized as prescribed by the physician.

10 *Spondylitis* is the inflammation of a vertebra. There are several types of spondylitis, all of which occur fairly infrequently. The types include ankylosing, rheumatoid, and traumatic spondylitis, spondylitis deformans, and Kummell's and Marie-Stumpell diseases. The nurse must be aware of the specific disease process in order to provide nursing care since each type has different ramifications. However, knowledge of the term spondylitis provides a clue as to the disease process. The nurse should seek in-depth information about the various types of spondylitis. Match the inflammatory condition with the most appropriate term.

b
e
d
c
a

_____ 1. Myositis   a. Tendon
_____ 2. Chondritis   b. Muscle
_____ 3. Synovitis   c. Vertebra
_____ 4. Spondylitis   d. Joint capsule
_____ 5. Tenosynovitis   e. Cartilage

11 Bursae are compartments that are filled with synovial fluid; the synovial compartments (or bursae) permit frictionless movement of bone and tissues over bony prominences. *Bursitis* is an inflammation of a bursa. Match the inflammatory condition with the appropriate phrase.

238

e	_____ 1. Chondritis	a. Joint capsule lining
d	_____ 2. Tenosynovitis	b. Inflamed muscle
b	_____ 3. Myositis	c. Vertebral inflammation
a	_____ 4. Synovitis	d. Tendon sheath inflammation
f	_____ 5. Bursitis	e. Inflamed cartilage
c	_____ 6. Spondylitis	f. Inflamed synovial compartment

12 The patient with bursitis complains of localized pain and tenderness, limited motion in the affected extremity, and possibly edema over the affected bursa. Bursae:

a, c, and d
a. Prevent friction
b. Prevent injury to the bones
c. Are compartments or sacs
d. Are filled with synovial fluid

13 As the inflammation progresses, the bursa may become filled with purulent material or calcium deposits, both of which are very painful for the patient. The symptoms of bursitis are (limited motion? pain? numbness? edema?).

limited motion, pain, edema

14 The nurse can alleviate the patient's discomfort by immobilizing the affected part and applying heat. On movement, the patient's pain becomes intense. Movement of the affected extremity is limited in bursitis because:

b
a. The bony prominences are inflamed
b. The bursa is no longer preventing friction
c. The purulent material creates edema

15 The physician may aspirate the purulent material from the bursa or surgically remove the calcium deposit. One of the most commonly affected bursae is the subdeltoid. Subdeltoid bursitis frequently requires surgery to remove calcium deposits. In addition to surgery, bursitis is also treated by _____ of the bursa.

aspiration

16 The physician may prescribe salicylates, phenylbutazone, or indomethacin for the treatment of bursitis. (These medications will be discussed later in this chapter.) The nursing care of the bursitis patient includes:

a, b, and d
a. Providing rest for the affected part
b. Supporting the affected part in a functional position
c. Removing the source of irritation from the bursa
d. Placing hot packs over the affected bursa

17 The aims of nursing care of the patient with the preceding inflammatory conditions include:

All of these
a. Preventing deformities

b. Providing relief from pain

c. Assisting the patient to function independently

18 *Osteomyelitis* is an infection of the bone that can be either acute or chronic. The bacteria entering an open wound, whether it is an open fracture or a surgical wound, or the bacteria from a systemic infection may be transported to a bone and produce an infection. Osteomyelitis is sometimes hematogenous. This means that infection is spread by _____ .

bloodstream

19 The femur, tibia, and humerus are the most common sites of osteomyelitis. The common element that describes the usual sites of osteomyelitis is that the involved bones are (short? long?).

long

20 *Staphylococcus aureus, Proteus, Pseudomonas,* and *Streptococcus* are the organisms most frequently identified as causing osteomyelitis. The treatment of acute osteomyelitis includes the administration of the appropriate antibiotic, as prescribed by the physician after blood and wound cultures have been taken. Blood cultures are taken to identify the causative organism because _____

the infection is systemic in origin

_____ .

21 Antibacterial agents may be administered parenterally in 50 to 300 ml of intravenous solution every 4 hours over a 4- to 6-week span. Parenteral therapy may be followed by a course of oral antibiotic therapy. The antibacterial agent to be administered depends on

the causative organism

_____ .

22 Until the causative agent has been specifically identified, the physician may prescribe nafcillin (Unipen), which is usually administered as 2 Gm. in 50 to 300 ml of 5% dextrose in water intravenously to be run in over 50 to 240 minutes. Treatment of the patient with osteomyelitis extends over a (long? short?) period of time.

long

23 In addition to nafcillin (Unipen), methicillin (Staphcillin), oxacillin (Keflin), or crystalline penicillin (intravenous) may be prescribed. These medications can be toxic to the vestibular or auditory branch of the cranial nerve or they may be nephrotoxic. Therefore the patient should be observed closely for _____

loss of hearing; dizziness; renal dysfunction

_____ , _____ , or _____

_____ .

24 The patient with acute osteomyelitis may be critically ill with a fulminating septicemia. Indicate which statements are true and which are false.

True	_____ a. Osteomyelitis is a preventable complication of bone surgery.
True	_____ b. Osteomyelitis may result from an infection in another part of the body.
False	_____ c. Osteomyelitis is a possible complication following a closed fracture.

25 During the acute phase of osteomyelitis, use of the affected part is usually prohibited since the bone is weakened and might fracture if submitted to stress. Complete each statement by filling in the blanks.

open

a. Osteomyelitis is a possible complication following a(n) _____ fracture.

after

b. Antibiotics are administered _____ a culture is obtained.

fracture

c. Osteomyelitis weakens the bone so that it might _____.

septic

d. In acute osteomyelitis, the patient is _____.

26 A splint, traction, or plaster cast may be utilized to provide rest for the affected part. When an extremity is put at rest by any of these

functional

methods, the position that is maintained must be _____.

27 Since the weakened bone might fracture if submitted to stress, the nurse must remember to support the affected limb as she moves it when giving care. Mr. Black has osteomyelitis of the right tibia. The nurse wants to move his right leg to the side of the bed to bathe

under the knee and the ankle or under the joints *(If you were unable to answer, review Section one.)*

it. The nurse should support his leg by placing the hands _____
_____
_____.

28 Although the infection may have been brought under control during the acute, septic phase of osteomyelitis, complete eradication of the bacteria is very difficult to attain because of the structure of bone. The organisms may continue to thrive in those portions of the bone that do not receive antibiotics by a direct blood supply; that is, the anatomic structure of bone makes it a barrier to drug penetration. List three antibiotics that may be used to treat osteomyelitis:

nafcillin; methicillin; oxacillin; cephalothin; crystalline penicillin *(any three, any order)*

_____, _____, or
_____.

29 If the patient receiving oxacillin has an elevated blood urea nitrogen or creatinine level, he should be watched closely for

renal dysfunction; possible toxicity

_____ and _____
_____.

30 A reduced rate of bone growth and muscle contractures are possible complications of osteomyelitis. Nursing actions therefore are directed toward prevention of the development of contractures as well as the prevention of other complications. The nurse, by putting the affected part at rest in a functional position, prevents

fractures; deformities _____ and _____.

31 In the chronic stage of osteomyelitis, the infection in the bone is dormant (inactive) for varying periods of time and then abruptly reactivates. During an exacerbation, purulent drainage accumulates at the infection site. A sinus tract develops to permit drainage, or the physician incises the site to permit drainage. Indicate which statements are true and which are false.

True _____ a. Osteomyelitis is difficult to cure.

False _____ b. The structure of bone does not influence the control of the bacteria.

True _____ c. Antibiotics are used in the treatment of osteomyelitis.

False _____ d. The blood supply transports the antibiotic to all parts of the bone.

32 As the infection progresses, small pieces of bone are often isolated from the remainder of the bone. The small pieces of bone are *sequestra*. Steps in treatment of osteomyelitis are:

b and d
a. Removal of the affected part
b. Control of the acute infection
c. Formation of sequestra
d. Drainage of the infection site

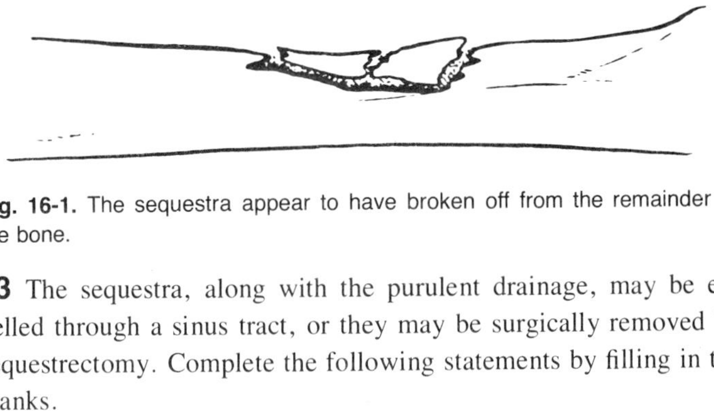

Fig. 16-1. The sequestra appear to have broken off from the remainder of the bone.

33 The sequestra, along with the purulent drainage, may be expelled through a sinus tract, or they may be surgically removed by sequestrectomy. Complete the following statements by filling in the blanks.

bone
a. Sequestra are pieces of _____.

progresses
b. Sequestra are formed as the infection _____.

isolated from
c. Sequestra are _____ the rest of the bone.

34 The surgeon often utilizes surgical procedures to remove the infection from the involved bone. *Saucerization* of the bone is the surgical removal of the scar tissue, the infected granulation tissue, and the sclerotic bone. Sequestrectomy is surgical removal of the

242

isolated pieces of bone,
sequestra

(scar tissue? isolated pieces of bone? sequestra? infected tissue?).

35 The physician may insert catheters at both ends of the wound after sequestrectomy and saucerization. The catheters are then used to irrigate and suction the wound postoperatively. Saucerization is performed to remove the (infection? infected granulation tissue? sclerotic bone? sequestra?).

infected granulation tissue,
sclerotic bone

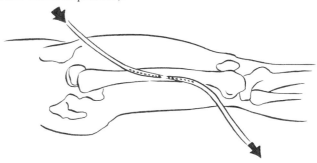

Fig. 16-2. Irrigation and drainage catheters after sequestrectomy and saucerization of osteomyelitis site.

36 Postoperatively, the nurse instills the antibiotic and/or detergent solution ordered by the physician into the catheter in the proximal end of the wound. The distal catheter is connected to a suction apparatus at the time(s) specified by the physician. Wound catheters are inserted:

a, b, d

a. To provide postoperative drainage
b. To allow the antibiotic solution to come into direct contact with the affected bone
c. To permit direct feeding of the bone
d. To permit suction of the wound

37 A plaster cast or a splint may be applied to the operated extremity after surgery if catheters are not inserted. A cast or splint is used to provide support to the weakened bone. The surgical procedures used in the treatment of osteomyelitis are _____

saucerization

sequestrectomy

and _____ .

38 The osteomyelitis patient often has numerous psychological problems that the nurse must help him to solve; these psychological problems may outnumber his physical nursing care problems. The psychological problems frequently stem from the chronic nature of the disease. As with other chronic conditions, the patient needs to understand and accept his diagnosis and to learn to function within his limitations. Which of the following psychological states tend to be associated with chronic diseases?

All of these
*(You should be able to
identify others also.)*

a. Depression   c. Anxiety
b. Hostility

39 The patient's anxiety may be related to his concern for the family's welfare, especially if he or she has been the main source of income for the family. Once the nurse has helped the patient to recognize and gain insight into the anxiety, the nurse may assist the patient in coping with the threat behind the anxiety. In situations such as this, the nurse's knowledge of community and hospital resources can be employed in helping the patient. Mr. White, 26 years old, has been admitted with a diagnosis of chronic osteomyelitis. (Mr. White sustained an open fracture of the right femur in an accident 2 years ago.) The nurse should talk with Mr. White:

All of these
a. To determine whether he is worrying about his family
b. To identify his psychological problems
c. To determine which diversionary activities would be appropriate

40 The principles of care of the patient in a cast are modified slightly if the cast has been applied to immobilize the part affected by osteomyelitis. The cast must be inspected routinely for evidence of drainage from the surgical wound. Drainage from the wound can saturate a plaster cast and weaken it, so that it must be handled with more care than usual. Observations of the extremity in a cast include

circulatory impairment; nerve damage; wound drainage

checking for _____,
_____, and _____
_____.

41 The physician frequently cuts a window in the cast so that the wound may be inspected and dressings changed. Postoperatively, Mr. White had a spica cast applied:

a, b, and d
a. To provide support for the femur
b. To immobilize the femur
c. To prevent spread of the infection
d. To prevent fracture of the right femur

42 Osteomyelitis is caused by bacteria that have entered the bone

a surgical wound; an open fracture; a systemic infection

by way of _____, _____
_____, or _____.

43 In acute osteomyelitis the critically ill patient is observed for

septic shock
signs of _____.

antibiotics
saucerization

44 Osteomyelitis is treated medically by administering _____
and surgically by (saucerization? cauterization?).

sinuses
sequestra

45 During the chronic phase of osteomyelitis, _____
and _____ are formed at the infection site.

pathological fracture; contrac-

46 Possible complications of osteomyelitis include _____

244

_____ , _____

_____ , _____

_____ , and _____ .

47 *Arthritis,* rather than being a specific disease entity, is a group of diseases and syndromes that have the common feature of joint involvement. Two types of arthritis are of particular interest in orthopedic nursing—*rheumatoid arthritis* and *osteoarthritis. Rheumatoid arthritis* is a chronic inflammation of the synovial lining of the joints. Currently, immune mechanisms, lysosomal enzymes, and viruses are being investigated as causative factors in rheumatoid arthritis, but no definite cause has been identified. The common characteristic of all types of arthritis is _____ .

48 Criteria have been established for determining the progression of the rheumatoid arthritis disease processes and for classifying the functional capacity of the rheumatoid arthritis patient. The nurse working routinely with arthritis patients should learn these criteria. As the disease progresses, the patient's functional capacity decreases as a result of the concomitant loss of joint mobility, muscle atrophy, and joint deformity. Indicate which statements are true:

a. Rheumatoid arthritis is a chronic, degenerative joint disorder.
b. Rheumatoid arthritis is an inflammatory disease of the joint synovial linings.
c. Rheumatoid arthritis is caused by an immune reaction.
d. Rheumatoid arthritis is a chronic inflammatory joint disease.

49 The rheumatoid arthritis patient experiences recurrent acute episodes, which are separated by periods of disease inactivity. These exacerbations and remissions, and their long-term effects on the patient's joints, comprise the chronic aspect of the disease. Periods of disease inactivity are called _____ ; acute disease episodes are called _____ .

50 The typical symptoms of acute rheumatoid arthritis are pain, swelling, heat, redness, and limited motion of the involved joints. During the acute phase, the patient may also experience malaise or fatigue and early morning joint stiffness. In acute rheumatoid arthritis the patient's involved joints are (fully functional? limited in motion?), (hot? normal?), (edematous? excoriated?), and (reddened? cyanotic?).

51 The physician's diagnosis is based on laboratory findings as well as symptoms. Mild anemia, an elevated erythrocyte sedimentation rate, and the presence of rheumatoid factor on a latex agglutination test are indicative of rheumatoid arthritis. During the initial acute episode roentgenograms are not usually taken because they tend to be inconclusive until the disease has progressed. The patient with rheumatoid arthritis usually has an elevated _____

erythrocyte sedimentation rate

_____ .

52 Mrs. Jones' admitting diagnosis is rheumatoid arthritis, and the nurse is making the admission assessment. If Mrs. Jones is experiencing an acute exacerbation, the symptoms the nurse would expect to observe are different from those that would be expected if the patient's disease is in remission. List the symptoms of acute rheumatoid arthritis.

a. Joint edema
b. Heat over involved joints
c. Redness of involved joints
d. Pain in involved joints
e. Limited joint motion
f. Malaise or fatigue
g. Early morning joint stiffness

a. _____

b. _____

c. _____

d. _____

e. _____

f. _____

g. _____

53 The physician often relies on nursing personnel, especially visiting nurses, to provide a thorough assessment of the patient. The assessment, laboratory tests, and clinical examination are integrated in establishing the diagnosis and selecting the method of treatment. Which of the following questions would be valuable to the nurse in assessing the extent and progression of Mrs. Jones' rheumatoid arthritis?

All of these

a. Can you bathe, feed, and dress yourself?
b. Can you do your own housework?
c. Do any of your joints occasionally "collapse"?
d. Have you been able to participate in your usual recreational activities?

54 As rheumatoid arthritis progresses, the joint structures are damaged by disease processes, such as scar tissue formation. Eventually the patient loses the use of the involved joints because of the resultant joint instability, deformity, malfunctioning, and fatigability. Prevention of joint damage is important since it can lead to joint (pain? disfiguration? instability? fatigability? engorgement? malfunction?).

disfiguration (deformity), instability, fatigability, malfunction

55 The muscle pull across the unstable joint, as the disease progresses, may cause flexion or extension contractures, subluxation, and/or joint dislocation. This process may eventually lead to ankylosis of the joint. In the acute phase of rheumatoid arthritis, medical therapy is focused on the relief of symptoms, especially pain, control of the inflammation, maintenance of function, and prevention

246

of joint deformity. Therefore, analgesic, anti-inflammatory, and antirheumatic drugs are prescribed. Medical therapy is directed

symptoms of pain
inflammation; function
joint deformity

toward relief of _____ , control of _____ , maintenance of _____ , and prevention of _____ .

56 The usual analgesic prescribed for the arthritic patient is aspirin. More potent analgesics, such as narcotics, are avoided since the chronic nature of rheumatoid arthritis will require continued administration and therefore presents a greater potential for addiction.

analgesic
(Their anti-inflammatory effect
in arthritis is controversial.)

Salicylates are recommended for the rheumatoid arthritis patient because of their _____ effect.

57 Numerous nonsteroid anti-inflammatory drugs, some of which are also analgesic and antipyretic, and now available for treatment of rheumatoid arthritis. Each of these medications has potential adverse effects; therefore the patient receiving one of them must be observed closely. The toxic reactions tend to be manifested in gastrointestinal, cutaneous, neurological, hematological, and/or cardiovascular side effects. Associate each of the following symptoms with the appropriate manifestation of toxicity.

c, e, g
b, d, h
a, l
i, k
f, j, m

_____ 1. Gastrointestinal   a. Skin rash
_____ 2. Hematological   b. Leukopenia
_____ 3. Cutaneous   c. Nausea
_____ 4. Cardiovascular   d. Anemia
_____ 5. Neurological   e. Vomiting
    f. Tinnitus
    g. Duodenal ulceration
    h. Thrombocytopenia
    i. Fluid retention
    j. Vertigo
    k. Sodium retention
    l. Urticaria
    m. Irritability

58 Table 1 lists the anti-inflammatory medications and the types of common adverse effects associated with each one.

59 List the reportable indicators of the following toxic reactions.

1. a. Nausea
   b. Vomiting
   c. Duodenal ulceration
2. a. Anemia
   b. Leukopenia
   c. Thrombocytopenia
3. a. Fluid retention
   b. Sodium retention

1. Gastrointestinal
   a. _____
   b. _____
   c. _____

2. Hematological
   a. _____
   b. _____
   c. _____

Table 1

| Drug | Possible adverse effects | | | | |
	Gastro-intestinal	Cuta-neous	Hema-tological	Cardio-vascular	Neuro-logical
Aspirin	X	X			X
Indomethacin (Indocin)	X	X	X	Fluid re-tention	X
Phenylbutazone (Butazolidin)	X	X	X	X	
Oxyphenbutazone (Tandoril)	X	X	X	X	
Fenoprofen (Nalfon)	X (rare)				
Ibuprofen (Motrin)	X (rare)				
Naproxen (Napnosyn)	X (rare)		Interacts with warfarin		
Tolmetin sodium (Tolectin)			Prolongs bleeding time	X Sodium retention	X

3. Cardiovascular

   a. _____

   b. _____

60 List the reportable indicators of the following toxic reactions to indomethacin.

1. Cutaneous

   a. _____

   b. _____

2. Neurological

   a. _____

   b. _____

   c. _____

1. a. Skin rash
   b. Urticaria
2. a. Vertigo
   b. Irritability
   c. Tinnitus

61 The antirheumatic compounds prescribed in the treatment of rheumatoid arthritis include chloroquine (Aralen), hydroxychloroquine (Plaquenil), gold salts (Myochrysine and Solganal), corticotropin (ACTH), and the synthetic adrenal corticosteroid hormones (prednisone and prednisolone), and cytotoxics and immunosuppressives (Imuran and Cytoxan). All of these medications can be extremely toxic, and they are prescribed only for the more advanced, severe stages of the disease. The nurse working with arthritic patients must continuously review and update knowledge regarding the antirheumatic and anti-inflammatory medications. Which of the following classes of medications is (are) used in the treatment of rheumatoid arthritis?

a, b, and e
(If you are unable to recall what uricosurics are used for, review Chapter 15.)

a. Antirheumatic agents
b. Anti-inflammatory agents
c. Uricosurics
d. Narcotics
e. Salicylates

62 Indicate whether the following drugs are (1) antirheumatic or (2) anti-inflammatory.

2	1	_____ Indocin	_____ Solganal
1	1	_____ Cytoxin	_____ Aralen
1	2	_____ ACTH	_____ Motrin
2	2	_____ Tolectin	_____ Naprosyn
2	1	_____ Butazolidin	_____ Prednisone

63 Nursing care goals for the rheumatoid arthritis patient should complement and supplement those of the medical plan. The initial nursing care goal for the newly admitted patient in an acute exacerbation is the same as that of the medical plan; the goal is to

relieve symptoms or pain

_____ .

64 This goal is not always easily attainable. The arthritis patient's pain forces him to seek a comfortable position, and once such a position is found, the patient tends to remain in it for extended periods of time. A comfortable position is not always beneficial; the patient may develop contractures, dysfunctional deformities, decubiti, and other complications. Nursing actions are taken to simultaneously

relieve pain; prevent complications

_____ and _____

_____ .

65 To relieve the pain, analgesics are administered as prescribed in conjunction with nursing measures. The patient's position must be closely supervised and the appropriate devices used to control his position. Positioning is important in the prevention of joint

contractures; deformities

_____ and _____ .

66 The rheumatoid arthritis patient frequently lies supine with his arms adducted and his elbows, wrists, hips, and knees flexed. If a large pillow is placed under his head, his neck is also flexed. Three devices that could be used to prevent the development of deformities

sandbags; pillows; rolled-up sheets or towels; arm splints (or any similar devices) *(any three, any order)*

are _____ , _____ , and _____ .

67 In addition to preventing deformities, the proper placement of these devices will _____

relieve the patient's pain or make the patient more comfortable

_____

_____ .

68 The arthritic patient may also develop flexion contractures of the spine and hips unless action is taken to prevent them. What supportive device would serve this purpose? _____

69 As the disease progresses, scar tissue forms in the joints, resulting in ankylosis, or stiffening, of the joints. Ankylosis is (joint subluxation? loss of joint motion? joint stiffness?).

70 With the progression of arthritis, ankylosis may not be preventable. If it occurs, the contractures that develop must be functional. For example, the fingers should be positioned so items can be grasped. The rheumatoid arthritis patient's contractures and deformities are the result of:

a. Pain and muscle spasms
b. Extended immobilization
c. The disease process
d. A dysfunctional position being continued over a long period of time

71 The patient's inflamed joints must have support both when at rest and when moved. When helping the patient to turn to his side, the nurse supports his legs by _____
_____ .

72 The rheumatoid arthritis patient who has had the disease for years may enter the hospital with joints that are already ankylosed. If flexion contractures of the knee joints are present, pillows should be placed under the joints to make the patient more comfortable. This is an application of the principle of:

a. Using all available means to prevent contractures
b. Supporting the joints at all times
c. Using nursing actions to prevent pain

73 Local applications of heat relieve pain and make the joints more supple, thus preparing the patient for exercises. The patient's extremities must be exercised to prevent disuse atrophy, improve muscle tone, and prevent _____ , _____ , or _____ .

74 Various types of heat applications are used on the rheumatoid arthritis patient, including warm moist compresses, whirlpool baths, and diathermy treatments. The resulting improved circulation to the joint:

a, b, and c

a. Relieves the patient's pain
b. Relaxes muscle spasms
c. Loosens the joints
d. Prevents the spread of infection

75 Passive, and later active, exercises are essential for the arthritis patient in order to:

a, b, and d

a. Prevent atrophy from lack of use
b. Prevent contractures
c. Prevent decubiti
d. Improve the tone of the muscles

76 Helping the patient and his family with psychosocial problems is one of the most important aspects in the nursing care of the rheumatoid arthritis patient. Personal and social adaptation to the disease is essential since this affects the patient's participation in and response to therapy. Adaptation has been defined as the process of changing behavior or performance in order to survive. Social adaptation, therefore, implies changing the way one interacts with others. The rheumatoid arthritis patient may need to change (his role in the family? his methods of communicating? his relationships with friends?).

All of these

77 The rheumatoid arthritis patient's relationships with his family and friends may be adversely affected by his condition, since the chronically ill patient often has difficulty maintaining his emotional health. The patient's pain and disability alter his need for communication, the message content of his communications, and his ego and body image. Assessment of the patient's psychological status is necessary to determine his degree of _____ and _____ adaptation.

personal
social

78 Which of the following statements would describe a poorly adapted rheumatoid arthritis patient?

All of these

a. He is anxious or depressed.
b. He lacks self-confidence
c. He feels insecure.
d. He hesitates to communicate his true feelings.
e. He is concerned about being a burden.

79 Which of the following nursing care goals are appropriate for the rheumatoid arthritis patient?

All of these
(c and d may result from immobility.)

a. To encourage the patient to do as much for himself as possible
b. To provide relief from pain
c. To prevent pneumonia and urinary stasis
d. To prevent deformities and contractures

e. To assist the patient in expressing his feelings about his condition

f. To assist the patient in understanding his condition and the methods of treatment

80 Which of the following nursing actions would be appropriate in the care of the rheumatoid arthritis patient?

a. Observe patient for indications of drug toxicity

b. Use supportive devices to maintain functional positions of all extremities

c. Implement appropriate psychotherapeutic measures

d. Interpret and reiterate information given by the physician

e. Identify patient's emotional state (denial, hostility, withdrawal, dependency, acceptance, etc.)

81 An arthroplasty or arthrodesis may be performed to correct the arthritis patient's deformities or to stabilize a joint to make it more functional. Knowledge of the availability of such procedures may provide encouragement to the patient, but it should be stressed that surgery does not obviate the need for continued, full, active participation in the medical treatment plan. The patient must accept the fact that his condition is (curable? treatable? acute? chronic?).

82 Total joint replacement has brought relief to many arthritic individuals. Some of these patients have had more than one joint replaced. However, it must be kept in mind that the long-range value of total joint replacement has not been established and the patient with rheumatoid arthritis may be young—the implication is that skilled nursing care to prevent deformity, muscle atrophy, or contractures is still a very essential part of the care of the arthritic person.

83 *Osteoarthritis* is a chronic, degenerative, noninflammatory disorder of the joints that is thought to be an inherent part of the aging process. Previous joint injury is often associated with the development of osteoarthritis. Match the disease with the phrase that completes the statement.

_____ 1. Rheumatoid arthritis

_____ 2. Osteoarthritis

a. Is chronic and crippling

b. Is chronic and degenerative

c. Is associated with the aging process

d. Has no known specific cause

e. Is an inflammatory disorder

84 As osteoarthritis progresses, the joints are gradually immobilized by fibrous contractures, and the patient begins having joint pain and stiffness. The patient usually notices the pain when moving the joint; joint stiffness is noticeable after periods of rest. Atrophy of the surrounding muscles may also be observed. The symptoms of osteoarthritis are joint _____ and _____ . The main symptoms of rheumatoid arthritis are joint _____ , _____ , _____ , _____ , and _____ .

85 Fewer joints are affected by osteoarthritis than by rheumatoid arthritis. The spine, hips, knees (the weight-bearing joints), elbows, and joints of the hand are commonly involved. When they are, the patient complains of joint pain and stiffness after _____ _____ and when _____ the joint.

86 The physician establishes the diagnosis of osteoarthritis on the basis of the patient's symptoms, the clinical examination, and x-ray studies of the involved joints. Match the diagnostic tools with the appropriate disease.

_____ 1. Rheumatoid arthritis   a. Clinical examination
_____ 2. Osteoarthritis   b. X-rays
                         c. Erythrocyte sedimentation rate
                         d. Blood count
                         e. Latex agglutination test

87 The medical therapy goals in the treatment of osteoarthritis are similar to those of rheumatoid arthritis. The therapeutic goals in osteoarthritis are to relieve pain, restore joint function, prevent disability, and control progression of the disease. The restoration of joint function is necessitated by the fact that the osteoarthritis patient tends to delay seeking medical care until the disease has progressed to the point where he is no longer able to function. The therapeutic goals in osteoarthritis are to:

a. _____
b. _____
c. _____
d. _____

88 The treatment of osteoarthritis includes the administration of aspirin and anti-inflammatory drugs such as phenylbutazone, resting the affected joints with appropriate support, applications of heat, exercise programs, and correction of abnormal posture. Each of these treatments is related to the medical therapy goals. Which of the treatments is (are) related to the goal of restoring joint function?

a. Administration of aspirin
b. Resting affected joints with support
c. Application of heat

253

d. Exercise

e. Correction of abnormal posture

89 The nursing care of the osteoarthritic patient is very much like that of the rheumatoid arthritis patient in terms of the physical aspects of care. Deformities and contractures are prevented in the same manner for the patient with osteoarthritis as for the patient with rheumatoid arthritis, but in osteoarthritis the joints involved are usually limited to:

a, c, and e

a. Fingers or hand

b. Feet or toes

c. Hips, knees, and ankle

d. Shoulders

e. Spinal column

90 The nurse should help the patient understand the disease process, particularly that osteoarthritis is *not* the same as rheumatoid arthritis. (Many osteoarthritic patients have misconceptions regarding the distinctions between the two.) The patient with osteoarthritis should be made comfortable using the techniques employed for the rheumatoid arthritis patient, such as:

a, b, c

a. Positioning him properly

b. Supporting the joints when he is moved

c. Using supportive devices

d. Administering narcotics and sedatives as prescribed

91 The patient with osteoarthritis does not have the severe pain and debilitating problems of the rheumatoid arthritis patient. The osteoarthritic patient should be encouraged to keep using the affected joints to prevent ankylosis and deformity. Exercises are beneficial in which of the following aspects?

a, b, and c

a. Muscle atrophy

b. Muscle spasms

c. Deformity correction

d. Disease prevention

92 Patients often believe there is a connection between arthritis and nutrition, but no relationship between the disease process and any particular type of diet has been substantiated. It is important for the obese patient with osteoarthritis to reduce his weight since it does put additional stress on the weight-bearing joints. Two important elements of nursing care of the osteoarthritic patient are

physical care; patient education

_____ and _____ _____ .

93 When the affected joint is edematous, the physician may opt to aspirate the fluid from the joint. Aspiration may be followed by intra-articular instillation of corticosteroids. It should be noted that this is usually the only use of corticosteroids for patients with osteoarthritis. Corticosteroids are prescribed for patients with

rheumatoid arthritis _____ .

94 The osteoarthritic patient's joints may continue to deteriorate in spite of treatment, and surgery may be indicated. An arthroplasty including total joint replacements will often relieve the patient's discomfort and improve joint motion. For some patients an arthrodesis or osteotomy may be selected by the physician as being the procedure that would be the most beneficial, although an arthrodesis relieves pain at the expense of loss of motion. The operative proce-

arthroplasty   dures employed in treatment of osteoarthritis are _____ ,

arthrodesis; osteotomy   _____ , and _____ .

95 A cast or traction may be applied to correct the osteoarthritic patient's deformities or to relieve pain. List the methods used to treat osteoarthritis.

a. Medications (aspirin) a. _____
b. Resting affected joint
   (supported)   b. _____
c. Applications of heat   c. _____
d. Exercise   d. _____
e. Surgery   e. _____
f. Cast   f. _____
g. Traction   g. _____
h. Correction of posture h. _____

96 Match the disease with the appropriate phrase.

a, b, c, d, f   _____ 1. Rheumatoid arthritis   a. Chronic condition

a, e, f   _____ 2. Osteoarthritis   b. Periods of remission

c. Debilitating with muscle atrophy

d. Widespread joint involvement

e. Limited to weight-bearing joints and hands

f. Joint pain and stiffness

97 The two types of arthritis that have been discussed are

rheumatoid arthritis   _____ and

osteoarthritis   _____ .

98 What characteristic do all forms of arthritis have in common?

joint involvement   _____ .

99 What are the symptoms of rheumatoid arthritis and osteoarthritis?

255

1. a. Joint edema
   b. Early morning joint stiffness
   c. Heat over involved joints
   d. Limited joint motion
   e. Malaise or fatigue
   f. Joint pain
   g. Redness of involved joints
   (any order)
2. a. Joint stiffness
   b. Joint pain

1. Rheumatoid arthritis
   a. _____
   b. _____
   c. _____
   d. _____
   e. _____
   f. _____
   g. _____
2. Osteoarthritis
   a. _____
   b. _____

ankylosed

100 As each disease progresses, the affected joints may become fibrosed or _____ .

101 List the types of medications prescribed in the treatment of rheumatoid arthritis.

a. Analgesics
b. Anti-inflammatory
c. Antirheumatic

a. _____
b. _____
c. _____

102 List the types of possible adverse side effects associated with anti-inflammatory drugs.

a. Gastrointestinal
b. Hematological
c. Neurological
d. Cutaneous
e. Cardiovascular

a. _____
b. _____
c. _____
d. _____
e. _____

103 List the symptoms associated with each of the following types of toxic reactions.

1. a. Nausea
   b. Vomiting
   c. Duodenal ulceration
2. a. Leukopenia
   b. Anemia
   c. Thrombocytopenia
3. a. Vertigo
   b. Irritability
   c. Tinnitus

1. Gastrointestinal complications
   a. _____
   b. _____
   c. _____
2. Hematological side effects
   a. _____
   b. _____
   c. _____
3. Neurological side effects
   a. _____
   b. _____
   c. _____

104 Briefly describe the anatomic structure affected by each of the following inflammatory conditions.

a. Synovial sheath of a tendon
b. Cartilage
c. Bones
d. Synovial lining of joint
e. Bursa(e)
f. Joint capsule lining

a. Tenosynovitis: _____

b. Chondritis: _____

c. Osteomyelitis: _____

d. Osteoarthritis: _____

e. Bursitis: _____

f. Synovitis: _____

105 Name two surgical procedures used in each of the following conditions:

1. a. Arthroplasty or total
      joint replacement
   b. Arthrodesis
   c. Osteotomy
      (any two, any order)
2. a. Sequestrectomy
   b. Saucerization
3. a. Arthroplasty or total
      joint replacement
   b. Arthrodesis

1. Osteoarthritis
   a. _____
   b. _____
2. Osteomyelitis
   a. _____
   b. _____
3. Rheumatoid arthritis
   a. _____
   b. _____

tenosynovitis; bursitis
rheumatoid arthritis

106 Three inflammatory conditions in which an application of heat is beneficial are _____ , _____ , and _____ .

osteomyelitis; rheumatoid
arthritis

107 Two inflammatory disorders in which the patient is prone to psychological problems requiring the nurse's assistance are _____ and _____ _____ .

The bursae are inflamed and
no longer prevent friction.

108 Briefly tell why the patient with bursitis experiences pain.

immobilizing the affected part;
applying heat to the
affected area

109 Two nursing actions taken to make the bursitis patient more comfortable are _____ _____ and _____ _____ .

aspiration of the purulent
material from the bursa;
surgical removal of calcium
deposits

110 Two methods of treating bursitis that are employed by the physician are _____ _____ and _____ _____ .

fractures; deformities

111 The patient with osteomyelitis requires nursing care to prevent _____ and/or _____ .

112 Describe what the nurse should check about each of the following points of the bedridden rheumatoid arthritis patient's position.

a. Neck: _____
b. Arms: _____
c. Legs: _____
d. Feet: _____

113 Many of the nursing actions employed in the care of the patient with rheumatoid arthritis accomplish two things at one time. These

measures _____ and

_____

_____ .

114 Match the term on the left with the appropriate phrase.

_____ 1. Tophi   a. Isolated pieces of bone
_____ 2. Sequestra   b. Stiffened fibrosed joints
_____ 3. Ankylosis   c. Urate salt deposits

115 Briefly describe the most common site of each of the following diseases.

a. Bursitis: _____

_____

b. Osteoarthritis: _____

_____

c. Gout: _____

_____

116 Periods of remission and exacerbation are typical of three

orthopedic conditions: _____ , _____

_____ , and _____ .

117 Before she administers any medication, the nurse is responsible for knowing:

a. The desired therapeutic effect of the drug
b. The toxic effects of the drug
c. The symptoms of toxicity
d. The normal dose of the drug

118 The chronically ill patient will need to learn how to live with

his disease; that is, he will need to _____ to it.

119 Arthritis is a (specific disease? group of diseases and syn-

dromes? specific syndrome?).

120 The nursing care goals of all patients with an inflammatory condition are similar. Two goals that would apply to almost any patient with an inflammatory condition include _____ _____ and _____ _____.

Suggested readings

Chapter 1

Hirschberg, G. G., Lewis, L., and Vaughn, P.: Promoting patient mobility, Nursing '77 **7**(5):42-46, May, 1977.

Kelly, M. M.: Exercises for bedfast patients, American Journal of Nursing **66**:2209-2213, Oct., 1966.

Smith, C.: Isometric exercises for men and women, Philadelphia, 1966, J. B. Lippincott Co.

Chapter 2

Brower, P., and Hicks, D.: Maintaining muscle function in patients on bed rest, American Journal of Nursing **72**:1250-1253, July, 1972.

Brown, M. L.: The quality of the work environment, American Journal of Nursing **75**:1755-1760, Oct., 1975.

Hoover, S. A.: Job-related back injuries in a hospital, American Journal of Nursing **73**:2078-2079, Dec., 1973.

Kamenetz, H. L.: Exercises for the elderly, American Journal of Nursing **72**:1401, Aug., 1972.

Long, B. C., and Buergin, P. S.: The pivot transfer, American Journal of Nursing **77**:980-982, June, 1977.

Millen, H. M.: Physically fit for nursing, American Journal of Nursing **70**:520-523, March, 1970.

Rantz, M. J., and Courtial, D.: Lifting, moving, and transferring patients, St. Louis, 1977, The C. V. Mosby Co.

Techniques for moving patients, Deerfield, Mass., 1976, Dray Publications, Inc.

Works, R. F.: Hints on lifting and pulling, American Journal of Nursing **72**:260-261, Feb., 1972.

Chapter 5

Birnstingl, M. A.: In Wilson, J. N., editor: Vascular injuries, fractures and joint injuries, New York, 1976, Churchill Livingston.

Donahoo, C.: Orthopedic neurovascular chart, Orthopedic Nurses Association Journal **4**(9):220-222, Sept., 1977.

Farrell, J.: Fat embolism syndrome, Orthopedic Nurses Association Journal **2**(2):41-42, 1975.

Glancy, G. L.: Compartment syndromes, Orthopedic Nurses Association Journal **2**(6):142-151, June, 1975.

Grimes, D. W., Garner, R. W., and Sorenson, N.: Origins of operative orthopedic infections, Orthopedic Nurses Association Journal **4**(5):144-146, May, 1977.

Iversen, L. D., and Clawson, D. K.: Manual of acute Orthopedic therapeutics, Boston, 1977, Little, Brown & Co.

Jones, V., and Killian, M.: Pulmonary embolism, Orthopedic Nurses Association Journal **2**(2):170-172, 1975.

Jones, V., and Killian, M.: Fat embolism syndrome, Orthopedic Nurses Association Journal **2**(2):41-42, Feb., 1975.

McFarland, M. D.: Fat embolism syndrome, American Journal of Nursing **76**(12):1942-1944, Dec., 1976.

Schoen, D. C.: Compartmental syndrome, Orthopedic Nurses Association Journal **4**(8):208-210, Aug., 1977.

Spickler, L.: Fat embolism, Orthopedic Nurses Association Journal **2**(6):146-147, June, 1975.

Whitesides, T. E., Harada, H., and Morimoto, K.: Compartment syndrome and the role of fastiotomy—its Parameters and techniques, Instructional Course Lectures **26**:174-176, 1977.

Chapter 6

Allgöwer, M., Matter, P., Perren, S. M., and Rüede, X.: The dynamic compression plate—DCP, New York, 1973, Springer-Verlag.

Clark, N.: Internal fixation of fractures using the basic principles of the Swiss study, Orthopedic Nurses Association Journal **3**(5):170-171, 1976.

Farrell, J.: Guidelines for nursing care of the elderly patient with a hip fracture and pinning, Warsaw, Ind., 1977, Zimmer. USA.

Hopson, H.: A simple method of treatment for humeral shaft fractures, Orthopedic Nurses Association Journal **3**(7):212-213, 1976.

Neufeld, A. J.: A ten-minute examination to pinpoint skeletal injuries, Orthopedic Nurses Association Journal **2**(11):273-274, 1975.

Ryan, J.: Compression in bone healing, American Journal of Nursing **74**:1998-1999, Nov., 1974.

Chapter 7

Anderson, M. G.: Orthopedic traction and nursing care, Orthopedic Nurses Association Journal **2**(12):304-307, Dec., 1975.

Brooks, H.: Cotrel or red rope traction, Orthopedic Nurses Association Journal **2**(7):173-174, July 1975.

Hogan, L., and Beland, J.: Cervical spine syndrome, American Journal of Nursing **76**(7):1104-1107, July, 1976.

Lewis, R. C.: Handbook of traction, casting and splinting techniques, Philadelphia, 1977, J. B. Lippincott Co.

Schmeisser, G.: A clinical manual of orthopedic traction techniques, Philadelphia, 1963, W. B. Saunders Co.

Stanley, K.: Swap and share: ortho seminar, Orthopedic Nurses Association Journal **1**(4):90, April, 1974.

The traction handbook, Warsaw, Ind., 1975, Zimmer. USA.

Twedt, B.: Skeletal traction for supracondylar fractures of

humerus, Orthopedic Nurses Association Journal 4(1): 9, Jan., 1977.

Chapter 8

Brown, R. E., and Preston, E.: Ambulatory treatment of femoral shaft fractures with a cast brace, Journal of Trauma 15:860, Oct., 1975.

Deyerle, W. M.: Broken legs are to be walked on, American Journal of Nursing 77(12):1927-1930, Dec., 1977.

Lewis, R. C.: Handbook of traction, casting and splinting techniques, Philadelphia, 1977, J. B. Lippincott Co.

Preto, A.: Patellar tendon bearing and cast braces: total contact orthoses in the weight-bearing treatment of tibial and femoral shaft fractures, Orthopedic Nurses Association Journal 4(1):10-11, Jan., 1977.

Weinheimer, P., and Blazevich, D.: Guidelines for cast care, Orthopedic Nurses Association Journal 2(6):138-139, 1975.

Chapter 9

Ackerman, S.: The orthopedic nursing diagnosis, Orthopedic Nurses Association Journal 2(2):58-59, March, 1975.

Alexander, M. M., and Brown, M. S.: Physical examination: the musculoskeletal system, Nursing '76 6(3):51-56, April, 1976.

Donahoo, C. A.: Orthopedic neurovascular chart, Orthopedic Nurses Association Journal 4(9):220-221, Sept., 1977.

Laird, M.: Techniques for teaching pre- and postoperative patients, American Journal of Nursing 75:1338-1340, Aug., 1975.

Malasanos, L., Barkauskas, V., Moss, M., and Stoltenberg-Allen, K.: Health assessment, St. Louis, 1977, The C. V. Mosby Co.

Neufeld, A. S.: A ten-minute examination to pinpoint skeletal injuries, Orthopedic Nurses Association Journal 2(11):273-274, Nov., 1975.

Roberts, S. L.: Skin assessment for color and temperature, American Journal of Nursing 75:610-613, April, 1975.

Snyder, M., and Baum, R.: Assessing station and gait, American Journal of Nursing 74:1256-1257, July, 1974.

Webb, K. J.: Early assessment of orthopedic injuries, American Journal of Nursing, 74:1048-1052, June, 1974.

Chapter 10

Ackerman, S.: The GSB total elbow, Orthopedic Nurses Association Journal 1(5):112-114, 1974.

Berger, M. R.: Dupuytren's contracture, American Journal of Nursing 78:244-245, Feb., 1978.

Hopson, H.: A simple method of treatment of humeral shaft fractures, Orthopedic Nurses Association Journal 3(7):212-213, July, 1976.

Inglis, A. E.: Total elbow joint replacement arthroplasty, Orthopedic Nurses Association Journal 4(8):211-214, Aug., 1977.

Volz, R. G.: Total wrist arthroplasty—a new surgical procedure, Orthopedic Nurses Association Journal 4(4):86-88, April, 1977.

Chapter 11

Aufranc, O. E., and Turner, R. H.: Total replacement of the arthritic hip, Hospital Practice 6:66-82, Oct., 1971.

Bennage, B., and Cummings, M.: Nursing the patient undergoing total hip arthroplasty, Nursing Clinics of North America 8(1):107-116, Mar., 1973.

Drain, C. B.: The athletic knee injury, American Journal of Nursing 71:536-537, Mar., 1971.

Eftekhar, N. S.: The infected total hip, Instructional Course Lectures 26:66-74, 1977.

Evarts, C. M., Amstultz, H. C., Riley, L. H., and Swanson, A. B.: Symposium on total joint replacement, Contemporary Surgery, June, 1974.

Eyre, M. K.: Total hip replacement, American Journal of Nursing 71:1384-1387, July, 1971.

Hamerton, E.: Management of total hip, femur, and knee replacement, Nursing Times 72:13, April, 1976.

Ishmael, W. K., and Shorbe, H. B.: Care of the feet, Philadelphia, 1967, J. B. Lippincott Co.

Ishmael, W. K., and Tkach, S.: Care of the knee, Philadelphia, 1977, J. B. Lippincott Co.

Johnson, C. F., and Convery, F. R.: Preventing emboli after total hip replacement, American Journal of Nursing 75:804-806, May, 1975.

Nelson, C. L.: Antibiotics in bone, joints and hematoma, Instructional Course Lectures 26:34-40, 1977.

Nute, L. F., and others: Nursing care of patients undergoing a total hip arthroplasty, Orthopedic Nurses Association Journal 3:43, Feb., 1976.

Poss, R., Ewald, F. C., Thomas, W. H., and Sledge, C. B.: Complications of total hip replacement arthroplasty in patients with rheumatoid arthritis, Journal of Bone and Joint Surgery 58(8):1130-1133, Dec., 1976.

Sculco, C. D., and Sculco, T. P.: Management of the patient with an infected total hip arthroplasty, American Journal of Nursing 75:584-588, April, 1976.

Shapiro, R.: Anticoagulant therapy, American Journal of Nursing 74:439-448, Mar., 1974.

Shirock, C.: Cast study: total knee replacement arthroplasty, Orthopedic Nurses Association Journal 4(7):179-186, July, 1977.

Staudt, A. R.: Femur replacement, American Journal of Nursing 75:1346-1348, Aug., 1975.

Thurston, E.: Orthopedic case study of a patient with a total hip arthroplasty, Orthopedic Nurses Association Journal 4(1):42-45, Feb., 1977.

Townley, C., and Hill, L.: Total knee replacement, American Journal of Nursing 74:1612-1617, Sept., 1974.

Chapter 12

Bount, W. P.: The non-operative management of scoliosis, Orthopedic Nurses Association Journal 3(1):19-21, 1976.

Bower, R. D.: Facet blocks; a new treatment for acute and recurrent backache, Orthopedic Nurses Association Journal 3(5):159-161, 1976.

Cailliet, R.: Low back pain syndrome, Philadelphia, 1968, F. A. Davis Co.

Cooper, S. B.: Low back pain caused by rupturing of the nucleus pulposus, Orthopedic Nurses Association Journal 2(9):224-230, 1975.

Dunn, B. H.: Scoliosis detection, Orthopedic Nurses Association Journal 2(11):282-283, 1975.

Finneson, B. E.: Low back pain, Philadelphia, 1973, J. B. Lippincott Co.

Ishmael, H. K., and Shrobe, H. A.: Care of the back, Philadelphia, 1969, J. B. Lippincott Co.

Kosuth, E.: Nursing care plan: anterior fusion for scoliosis, Orthopedic Nurses Association Journal 1(5):115, 1974.

Marcus, W. E.: Fractures and dislocation of the spine, Orthopedic Nurses Association Journal 1(4):94-95, 1974.

Matzka, L.: Nursing care—scoliosis surgery, Orthopedic Nurses Association Journal 2(10):251-255, 1975.

Mooney, V., Cairns, D., and Robertson, J.: The psychological evaluation and treatment of the chronic back pain patient—a new approach, Orthopedic Nurses Association Journal 2(7):163-165, 1975; 2(8):187-189, 1975.

O'Connor, B. J.: Scoliosis: classification and diagnosis, Orthopedic Nurses Association Journal 3(3):84-88, 1976.

Viray, P. C.: Nursing care of the patient with a cervical spine injury, Orthopedic Nurses Association Journal 2(5):115-118, 1975.

Wells, R. E.: Lumbar laminectomy and/or fusions, Orthopedic Nurses Association Journal 1(2):33-36, 1974.

Chapter 13

Barnes, G. H., and Levy, S. W.: Stump edema, Washington, D. C., The American Orthotics and Prosthetics Association.

Brady, E.: Grief and amputation, American Nurses Association Clinical Sessions, New York, 1968, Appleton-Century-Crofts.

Buck, B., and Lee, A. D.: Amputation: two views, Nursing Clinics of North America 11(4):641-657, Dec., 1976.

Engstrand, J. L.: Rehabilitation of the patient with a lower extremity amputation, Nursing Clinics of North America 11(4):659-670, Dec., 1976.

Levy, S. W., and Barnes, G. H.: Stump hygiene, San Francisco, University of California School of Medicine.

McClinton, V. S.: Nursing of the upper extremity amputee and preparation for prosthetic training, Nursing Clinics of North America 11(4):671-678, Dec., 1976.

Melzack, R.: Phantom limbs, Psychology Today 4:63-68, Oct., 1970.

Pasnau, R. D., and Pfefferbaum, B.: Psychological aspects of post-amputation pain, Nursing Clinics of North America 11(4):679-686, Dec., 1976.

Pfefferbaum, B., and Pasnau, R. D.: Amputation grief, Nursing Clinics of North America 11(4):687-690, Oct., 1976.

Chapter 14

Graber, E. A., and Barber, H. R.: The case for and against estrogen therapy, American Journal of Nursing 75:1766-1771, Oct., 1975.

Hermann, I. F., and Smith, R. T.: Gout and gouty arthritis, American Journal of Nursing 64:111-113, Dec., 1964.

Robinson, C. H., and Lawler, M. R.: Normal and therapeutic nutrition, New York, 1977, Macmillan, Inc.

Rodnan, G. P., editor: Gout; Primer on the Rheumatic Diseases, ed. 7, New York, 1973, The Arthritis Foundation.

Soika, C. V.: Combating osteoporosis, American Journal of Nursing 73:1193-1197, July, 1973.

Chapter 15

Webb, K. J.: Early assessment of orthopedic injuries, American Journal of Nursing 74:1048-1052, June, 1974.

Chapter 16

Anxiety recognition and interventions (programmed instruction), American Journal of Nursing 65:129-152, Sept., 1965.

Ehrlich, G. E., editor: Total management of the arthritic patient. Philadelphia, 1973, J. B. Lippincott Co.

Hoffman, A. L.: Psychological factors associated with rheumatoid arthritis, Nursing Research 23:218-234, May-June, 1974.

Klinger, J. L.: Self-help manual for arthritis patients, New York, 1974, The Arthritis Foundation.

Loxley, A. K.: The emotional toll of crippling deformity, American Journal of Nursing 72:1839-1840, Oct., 1972.

MacGinniss, O.: Rheumatoid arthritis—my tutor, American Journal of Nursing 68:1699-1701, Aug., 1968.

Medical and Scientific Committee, The Arthritis Foundation: Manual for nurses, physical therapists, and medical social workers, New York, The Arthritis Foundation.

O'Dell, A. S.: Hot packs for morning-joint stiffness, American Journal of Nursing 75:986-987, June, 1975.

Prilook, M. E.: Calcific tendinitis and bursitis, Patient Care, pp. 18-33, Aug. 15, 1972.

Rodnan, G. P., editor: Primer on the rheumatic diseases, New York, 1973, The Arthritis Foundation. Available on request from the Arthritis Foundation.

General

Aegerter, E., and Kirkpatrick, J. A.: Orthopedic disease, Philadelphia, 1975, W. B. Saunders Co.

Blauvelt, C. T., and Nelson, F. R. T.: A manual of orthopedic terminology, St. Louis, 1977, The C. V. Mosby Co.

Brigham, L.: Radiological procedures in orthopedics, Orthopedic Nurses Association Journal 4(7):164-168, 1977.

Donahoo, C. A., and Dimon, J. H.: Orthopedic Nursing, Boston, 1977, Little, Brown & Co.

Farrell, J.: Illustrated guide to orthopedic nursing, Philadelphia, 1977, J. B. Lippincott Co.

Hirschberg, G. G., Lewis, L., and Vaughn, P.: Rehabilitation: a manual for the care of the disabled and elderly, Philadelphia, 1976, J. B. Lippincott Co.

Jones, S. L.: Orthopedic injuries: illness as deviance, American Journal of Nursing 75:2030-2033, Nov., 1975.

Kavchak-Keyes, M. A.: Four proven steps for preventing decubitus ulcers, Nursing '77 7:58-61, Sept., 1977.

Kerr, A.: Orthopedic nursing procedures, New York, 1969, Springer Publishing Co.

Larson, C. B., and Gould, M.: Orthopedic nursing, St. Louis, 1974, The C. V. Mosby Co.

Malasanos, L., Barkauskas, V., Moss, M., and Stolten-berg-Allen, K.: Health assessment, St. Louis, 1977, The C. V. Mosby Co.

McCaffery, M.: Nursing management of the patient with pain, Philadelphia, 1972, J. B. Lippincott Co.

Neimark, R. G.: A doctor discusses care of the back, Chicago, 1976, Budlong Press.

Pace, J. B.: Pain; a personal experience, Chicago, 1976, Nelson-Hall Co.

Powell, M.: Orthopedic nursing, London, 1977, Churchill Livingston.

Roaf, R., and Hodkinson, L. J.: Textbook of orthopedic nursing, London, 1975, Blackwell Scientific Publications.

Schneider, F. R.: Handbook for the orthopedic assistant, St. Louis, 1976, The C. V. Mosby Co.

Sine, R. D., Liss, S. E., Roush, R. E., and Holcomb, J. D.: Basic rehabilitation techniques, Germantown, Md., 1977, Aspen Systems Corp.

263